7 Simple Steps to a Healthier You

Dawn Hall

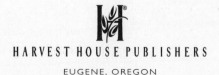

HARVEST HOUSE PUBLISHERS

EUGENE, OREGON

Scripture quotations are taken from the HOLY BIBLE, NEW INTERNATIONAL VERSION®. NIV®. Copyright©1973, 1978, 1984 by the International Bible Society. Used by permission of Zondervan. All rights reserved.

Cover by Terry Dugan Design, Minneapolis, Minnesota

Cover photos © Burke/Triolo Productions / Brand X Pictures / Getty Images; Rubberball / Rubberball Productions / Getty Images; Peter Scholey / Photographer's Choice / Getty Images; BananaStock / Alamy; Tetra Images / Alamy; Stockbyte Platinum / Alamy

Published in association with the literary agency of Allen O'Shea Literary Agency LLC, 615 Westover Road, Stamford, CT 06902

Readers are advised to consult with their physician or other medical practitioner before implementing the suggestions that follow. This book is not intended to take the place of sound medical advice. Neither the author nor the publisher assumes any liability for possible adverse consequences as a result of the information contained herein.

7 SIMPLE STEPS TO A HEALTHIER YOU
Copyright © 2006 by Dawn Hall
Published by Harvest House Publishers
Eugene, Oregon 97402

Library of Congress Cataloging-in-Publication Data
Hall, Dawn.
7 simple steps to a healthier you / Dawn Hall.
p. cm.
ISBN-13: 978–0-7369–1335–5 (pbk.)
ISBN-10: 0–7369–1335–1
1. Health—Religious aspects—Christianity. I. Title: Seven simple steps to a healthier you. II. Title.
BT732.H333 2006
241.'68—dc22   2005027588

Printed in the United States of America

06 07 08 09 10 11 12 13 14 / BP-MS / 10 9 8 7 6 5 4 3 2 1

Contents

Introduction

I gave God many excuses why I should not write this book. "Now isn't a good time." "I know what to do, but I am not sure I have the discipline right now." "I could do it later." "What if I fail or have to quit?"

These all sounded vaguely familiar.

It took me a few days to realize that this list of excuses was familiar because it is the same list I used for years to avoid stepping into a life of proper diet and exercise. Isn't it amazing how our fears of weakness resurface wearing different disguises? Here I thought I was reasonably evaluating whether to create this book, when all along I was sifting through recycled thoughts.

Once I recognized this, I knew what I had to do and what I had to offer. I have been there. At times I still struggle to be healthy. I understand that our personal journey to health and fitness can seem nearly impossible, especially while leading a busy life. If you are like me, one of the top excuses on the list is that you just don't have time to evaluate your eating, go for walks, and "manage" your weight and health. You are probably managing a job, a home, a family, or any combination of these.

That should be enough.

But it isn't. You do need more. You need to know that your journey is not fruitless and that there is a way through excuses and obstacles to a life that offers strength, health, satisfaction, and fulfillment.

My Story—I Was Born Watching My Weight

I am the oldest of seven children. I grew up with very unhealthy eating patterns. I was always the largest in my classes growing up. In part because I got held back in first grade, making me a year older than my classmates, and also in part because I have a large frame.

My stepfather raised cattle, chickens, and rabbits and kept a garden. We took pride in how much we could eat. *You can eat six ears of corn? I can eat seven. You can eat five pieces of pizza? I can eat six.* Our ideas of healthy eating were all about quantity and competition.

When I was 15 I rode my bike about five miles to McDonald's every day and worked as a hostess and behind the counter. I loved that job. Because I was riding my bike back and forth to work daily, I didn't think I needed to be concerned with the quantity of free meals I was consuming. I gained 18 pounds during summer break. As a cheerleader, this kind of weight gain was my biggest fear. So I did what countless women do when faced with their unhealthy choices; I made even *unhealthier* choices. I skipped breakfast, ate only a small salad for lunch, skipped dinner, and ate two or three pieces of carob in the evening after working out.

I struggled with those stubborn 18 pounds throughout high school and ate minimal food the last few months before graduating in order to look good at my graduation party. I was always hungry and tired.

Then years later came the births of my two girls. These were especially joyous occasions because there was a point when I thought I would not be able to have children. However, in my continued unhealthy state of being, I tainted these happy events by worrying about my weight during my pregnancies.

I have always had a preoccupation with food, thoughts of food, and an underlying desire to eat sweets. It wasn't until I went on the Atkins diet and later the South Beach diet that I realized part of the reason I crave and eat sweets is because I am a carbohydrate junkie. Sugar is my fix. While my cravings did not disappear on these diets, they were less intense than when I eat carbohydrates such as white flour, refined sugar, and other processed foods.

When low fat became more prevalent, this fueled my creativity all the more...and it suited my goal at the time to lose weight. I tried out new ideas for dinner and then the next day I would take the leftovers to my aerobic students and W.O.W. (Watching Our Weight) group. "You should write a cookbook," I heard over and over again from my students who loved the recipes. Eventually I did. Several of them. And they were all born out of a desire to find ways to eat healthy and hearty without gaining weight.

When it comes to our weaknesses, we can either be bitter or better. We can hold on to our inadequacies or we can let God help us and use us one day at a time. My passion for food wasn't a curse after all. God used it for good.

Later in this book I will discuss how spiritual fitness directly relates to, affects, and supports physical and emotional fitness. Because of the significance of all three areas, in each chapter I offer ideas to connect you to physical, emotional, and spiritual health. It is when we invest in all of these areas that our vision of health can be realized.

Your Story

My hope is to provide you with easy-to-manage tools to shape your choices for a lifetime rather than just adjust your eating habits for a short period of time. As you turn toward healthier living, you will weed out behaviors or ideas that undermine your effort.

Of course, the choice is all yours. But once you have made the decision, I am here for you. I strongly believe we can discover a simple, healthy plan for each of our lives. We may be blessed with gifts of abundant health, love, joy, peace, and prosperity, but we also have to do our part. The gift of good health is intended for us, but we have to open the beautiful package, put it on, wear it, and use it. Whether this gift is utilized or not is up to you. The gift of good health is a gift only you can give yourself.

It is not easy to be obedient and willing to receive the gift of good health. It is not easy to ignore excuses that ring out in our heads and sabotage our hard work. But it is well worth the *priceless* gifts of love, joy, peace, serenity, and strength we receive in return.

My guess is that you are a busy person who is tired of wasting precious time on efforts that yield little. If that is the case, let's not waste one more moment of your journey.

_____ **The Satisfied Life**

When we start down the road to better health, we often are limping along or even wandering away from good choices. We feel anything but satisfied with ourselves and our circumstances. This process of looking at your own story and reshaping your body, mind, and spirit will provide an amazing side effect—you will discover satisfaction. You will get to a place where perfection is not the goal; rather, progress is what you seek. We will look at what makes up the satisfied life. You might discover that you have had the ingredients all along. Some of us might see elements we have been missing. And still others will not be ready to see what they need. But if you are ready to begin, a life of satisfaction and fulfillment is just around the bend.

Devotional Health

How have you felt about your story up until now? How would you talk about the beginning of your story? The middle? The present chapter? How many chapters have you spent on worrying about your weight? Let's move toward the desire for peace and contentment, and this will be a new experience. Take time today or this week to think about how you might want your story to change. What does this new chapter look like? Feel like? Write your answers in the back of this book in the journal provided for you.

Prayer

God, give me strength to become a healthy, strong, and fulfilled person. May I seek Your guidance and Your measure of my worth as I take the steps necessary to change my health for the better. Let me use my progress to glorify and serve You. Amen.

Shaping Tools

For your journey through the *7 Simple Steps to a Healthier You*, I recommend the following tools be gathered and used over the course of the next days, weeks, or months—depending on the timeline you have set for yourself to work through this book.

Tool 1: Journal. Each of the seven steps will have midstep assessment questions that can be answered either in this book or in your journal. Also, the Devotional Health reflections, questions, and suggestions are perfect starters for your journal entries during this process. My hope is that you will use your journal as a support for healthier living in the years to come. If you don't pick one up right away, I have some journal pages at the back of this book to get you started.

Tool 2: Nutrition reference book. Choose one with nutrition information for lots of foods.

Tool 3: Reusable bottle for drinking water. Start this process right. Be sure to get enough water every step of the way.

Tool 4: Contentment scale. Hide your bathroom scale and do not weigh yourself more than once a week. Our goal is overall good health. Our daily focus is on being healthy, not on what we weigh. As we focus on the core of what is important— living healthily—the rewards of losing excess body fat will naturally happen. We will become leaner, more toned, and healthier in *all* aspects of our life. I suggest taking a piece of paper and drawing the outline of a real bathroom scale on it. Inside that outline, write the following measures of contentment:

I feel...

1. Down about life
2. Frustrated, but I know this is temporary
3. Content with myself and the process
4. Pleased with how I am doing and with my attitude
5. Excited about life and my commitment to a healthier me

When you make an entry in your journal, indicate how you "weigh in" on the contentment scale. This is one time when you will be excited to see the numbers go up. And this is a reminder that your real success is not a measurement of weight lost, but of contentment and peace gained.

Make the Choice

The beginning of any race or effort has a starting line. This race begins at the starting line called "choice." To prepare for the following seven simple steps to a healthier you, examine what the important choice for success is, how to make it, and how to keep it.

"Am I ready to see my desire for a healthier life realized?"

This is a good question to define your choice. We could consider it a simple yes or no question, but for any of us who have tried to move toward healthier living a time or two in the past, we know this is not simple.

But it can be done.

The key to wholeness of mind, body, spirit, health, and prosperity is making a conscious choice. If we commit only halfway to this effort, the results will never be lasting and our behavior, heart, and lifestyle will not be changed. Desire without action—without follow-through—is useless.

Are you at a place along your journey where you are willing to exchange potentially negative decisions that steal your energy for choices that boost your energy and inspiration? If so, the rewards are abundant and lasting. Look at each choice or sacrifice with a positive rather than negative attitude. Instead of thinking about what you are giving up, think of the tremendous rewards and benefits you will be getting. A bag of chips and low self-esteem in exchange for great health and a body you'll feel good in is a great exchange.

If you are not fully satisfied in any one area of your life, then you are not living at your fullest potential. For example, it is not God's desire for you to have a strong marriage and terrific children and yet be in such poor health that you cannot enjoy simple pleasures with them, such as a bike ride or a long walk in the park. It is not God's desire for you to please everyone in your life all the time and yet sacrifice your energy, peace, and potential.

When we choose an unhealthy lifestyle, we are subconsciously saying to ourselves, *I am not worth the time, energy, or effort it takes to be who I want to be.*

I used to be so obsessed about not eating (even though I was constantly craving food) that I even went so far as to tell my husband what I had eaten throughout the day. I would report to him after he'd come home from work. I was looking for affirmation, but he never understood why I felt compelled to share this information. I'll never forget how crushed I was when he told me, "Honey, why do you tell me what you eat?" *Isn't he proud of me? Can't he see how hard I am trying?*

My view of health was so distorted that I blended my hunger for affirmation with food. I had not yet made the choice to commit to healthy living. I was living a double life by saying I wanted to be fit and active and yet making choices that were not in favor of health. They were about deprivation, sacrifice, and self-punishment. I didn't understand I was supposed to give myself grace and support. I wasn't on my own side, so I wanted my husband to lavish praises for good behavior onto me as soon as he came home. No wonder it became a vicious cycle of defeat in those days. One minute I was acting like a child sneaking food, and the next moment I was the disapproving parent chastising the child for breaking the rules and ruining the chance for success.

The moment you make the decision and the commitment to become healthier, you have become the new and improved you. Just like that. New self-confidence, inner peace, and a healthier physical appearance are your rewards. They are the evidence that you are committed to being your number one supporter. Once you make the choice, you are well on your way. This time really will be different.

Instant Gratification or Instant Gratitude

Wouldn't it be fantastic to be instantly transformed physically? We could sit back, munching our favorite junk food, and think things into existence rather than putting in the work or effort.

The only problem with this scenario is that we would miss the true transformation that takes place during the journey. We would miss the incredible gifts that are meant to be a part of this adventure called life. Some of these gifts include:

awareness	commitment
knowledge	hope
peace	renewal
understanding	growth
self-confidence	

I'm sure you can think of many other gifts you have received when you have given something your all. Chances are you made a big effort on someone else's behalf. For many of us, this is our strength. But when we turn the effort toward our own lives, we often struggle.

As you make your choice for you, for your health, for a life of goodness and significance, you will face many little choices. And you will discover that the real choice will be between instant gratification and instant gratitude. An example...you find you have a rare hour of free time during the early evening. You consider going for a walk around the neighborhood or watching a television show you have seen a few times. Neither is a wrong choice, but one leans more toward instant gratification (television) and one leans more toward instant gratitude.

Gratification feels good but doesn't always support long-term wellness—and often it is followed by inklings of remorse. Though we are given all-encompassing grace from God, we are still creatures of regret. This is such a strong part of our destructive nature that some people become bitter and never get past their choices.

Gratitude comes with appreciation for making or receiving a healthy choice. The wellness resonates from a deeply spiritual place. And I would bet that if you chose to walk around the neighborhood, a sense of healthy gratification would also be a part of that experience.

Deliberately make a choice and see which decision will lead you to gratitude, if not in the moment, then later on as you enjoy the benefits of healthy patterns and habits.

Renewal Begins by Renewing Your Mind

A change in lifestyle is one of the surest ways to realize how much faulty thinking is ruling or ruining your health. For years you might not have noticed your "one step forward, two steps back" routine, but when you incorporate change, you start realizing past mistakes.

When this awareness comes—and believe me, it will—it is time to put in the work of renewing your thoughts so that new behaviors, actions, and decisions will take shape. In Scripture we are given the secret to this difficult endeavor: "Do not conform any longer to the pattern of this world, but be transformed by the renewing of your mind. Then you will be able to test and approve what God's will is—his good, pleasing and perfect will" (Romans 12:2).

We will explore the key directives in this verse that will inspire a new way of thinking and living.

Do Not Conform to the Pattern of This World

Even if you have not been on a program or consciously thinking through what you eat or how active you are, you have chosen a philosophy about how to treat your body. The old "decision by indecision" practice of default is a very popular choice.

How do you allow the patterns of the world or the patterns of indifference rule your health? Let's identify some of the familiar ways this happens for many of us:

- We allow fast food or fatty food to become our primary nutrition.

- Convenience dictates the pace and substance of our day.

- Trends tempt us to embrace unhealthy habits.

- We look to the bodies of others to measure our own health.

- Cultural priorities determine our spiritual, emotional, and physical direction.

Patterns of the world can rule our hearts and bodies from an early age. How many of us looked at our classmates in grade school and noticed differences that left us worried, anxious, or sad? Whatever the differences—economics, body types, talents, personalities—we noticed. And in our minds we tucked away that bit of jealousy or fear or self-destructive doubt and traded God's pure view of our lives for our newly skewed one.

As we reject the pattern of this world and make the choice to get healthy, to treat ourselves with respect, and to honor God's view of our bodies and selves, we must follow the next step. We renew our minds.

Be Transformed by the Renewing of Your Mind

When you see "renewing your mind," is your first thought "Easier said than done"? Well, I have good news for you. What is *said*—to ourselves and to others—can impact the renewing of our minds. The language that flows into our minds, through our hearts, and out of our mouths shapes our thoughts and actions.

Let's revisit the list from the previous section and allow a different thought process to direct it. Think on these from a new perspective and philosophy. Try each one.

- We allow fast food or fatty food to become our primary nutrition.

    Quickly prepared, healthy food will be more valuable to our bodies.

- Convenience dictates the pace and substance of our day.

> *Commitment moves us toward good, conscious choices day and night.*

- Trends tempt us to embrace unhealthy habits.

> *A steadfast plan keeps us on track with healthy habits.*

- We look to the bodies of others to measure our own health.

> *Looking to God for validation gives us a loving measure of ourselves.*

- Cultural priorities determine our spiritual, emotional, and physical direction.

> *Personal healthy priorities keep us on a consistent path that leads to whole health.*

What language do you use to discuss your own body? Do terms like "fat" or "old" or "worn out" pop out of your mouth? Try discussing your body in more positive terms. If you are in need of losing weight, consider your body "ready for exercise and change." When you feel the aches and pains of age or body misuse, say, "My body is asking for help."

Be your body's best friend and advocate. When you have a free hour in your day, you could sit in a coffee shop with a scone and a latte as your break from the day's pace or you could exercise. Consider which choice best serves your body, which choice could lead to a new, improved habit. And just as the exercise will build your strength and stamina, there will certainly be times when that coffee shop scenario will also be a source of mental health. It becomes a balancing act.

Stand up for your body and your goals. Transform the way

you treat the legs that carry you home or to work, the arms that hold your children and hug your spouse, the mind that provides you with ideas and inspiration.

Ready for Success

I have observed there are key significant factors in all individuals who successfully are obtaining and maintaining their healthier lifestyles:

1. Something clicks inside and they have a desire to change for the better (healthier), but it is more than just a desire. They are willing to do whatever it takes so they can be the more fulfilled person they know God intends them to be.

2. They eat healthy food they enjoy.

3. The exercise plan they choose is not something they think of as drudgery; it is something they enjoy.

4. They have accountability—at least one person to whom they are accountable.

5. The healthier change is a transformation from the inside out.

To renew your way of thinking and living, it helps to have a plan. We discover our plan best when we have evaluated our goals. The seven simple steps in this book will serve you and your health best if you invest in the evaluation, reflection, and observation exercises in each chapter. The following questions will move us from considering a change to pursuing a change.

What is your goal?

Why do you want to achieve this goal?

Do a painfully honest appraisal of yourself. What has held you back in the past from not successfully attaining and maintaining your goal? (If you cannot identify these things yet, you will be able to in later chapters.)

How will you keep these same things from hurting your goal this time?

Replace old unhealthy thinking patterns with healthy thoughts. What are some of your biggest mental hang-ups? What are the negative or destructive thoughts which rule your health?

List ten unhealthy eating patterns you struggle with and then follow it with at least one positive replacement thought or action.

Example: *I love sweets, but they leave me craving more sugar. When I eat fruit and vegetables, they fill me up and provide nutrients.*

1.

2.

3.

4.

5.

6.

7.

8.

9.

10.

Initially you may have to do what I call "fake it till you make it." Remember, what you think about, you bring about. Trust me, with time you will begin to feel what your head and heart have known all along as truth.

If you are at a place in your life where self-discipline is something totally out of character for you, then you need to be up-front and honest with yourself that self-discipline is not something you are accustomed to. Honesty with yourself is the best policy. In order for you to move forward, you need to know and acknowledge to yourself and to God your areas of weakness (also known as character flaws). Knowledge is power. As you learn to be honest with yourself, you can accept your flaws and strengths. Give them over to God. Ask for and receive His help.

List ten self-defeating mind games you struggle with that hold you back from obtaining or maintaining your goals. After you write each one down, next to it write at least one positive replacement thought you will now choose to replace old thinking.

Example: *Until I lose weight, I am unhappy. At every weight, I will be glad about my efforts to living healthier.*

1.

2.

3.

4.

5.

6.

7.

8.

9.

10.

The first step to wholeness of mind, body, spirit, health, and prosperity is choosing to obey. We need to make a conscious choice. Desire without action is useless. I don't care how much we say we want something, if we are not willing to do what we have to do to get the results, then we don't want it badly enough.

So let me ask you, what price are you willing to pay for terrific health, serenity, prosperity, love, joy, and peace? Are you willing to exchange one hour of sitting on the couch for one hour of walking three times a week to have the body you want, or is the price not worth it? The rewards are abundant and overflowing. Think of the price you pay as a gift you give yourself. Look at it with a positive attitude instead of a negative. Instead of thinking what you are giving up, think of the tremendous rewards and benefits you will be receiving. When was the last time you felt good about you?

The Satisfied Life

Many of us face our troubles by either eating or neglecting ourselves. It seems a strange way to really address our worries or concerns, but somewhere along the way we learned that stuffing down our problems was better than seeking satisfaction. Your path now is about finding true satisfaction and fulfillment in your daily living. It is possible. It is attainable. And it is happening. Right here, right now in your life.

Begin this quest for satisfaction by allowing yourself to feel the emotions tied to eating and exercising. No more stuffing the feelings or the food. And no more stifling your needs and dreams. It is time to discover exactly who you are when you are not worried about weight or meeting the demands of everybody in your life. This journey is not a free pass to a life of no responsibility, but it is a journey that begins with responsibility to the *you* God made. This is the way of satisfaction.

Devotional Health

Meditate on the following verse from Jeremiah. In your journal or in the space below the verse, describe what it means to you to have a hope, a future, and a plan. As you begin to discover how to be healthier, what emotions are strongest? What is your hope for your plan to get healthy?

"For I know the plans I have for you," declares the LORD, "plans to prosper you and not to harm you, plans to give you hope and a future" (Jeremiah 29:11).

Prayer

God, help me let go of the negative things in my life that I hold on to. Show me Your purpose for my life and guide my steps as I seek Your strength to become stronger, healthier, and more grounded. Amen.

Step 1 | Set Yourself Up for Success

Was there a point in time when you stopped caring for yourself? For some this started in childhood, when unhealthy behaviors were modeled by parents or family members. For others it began when they became wives and mothers and the responsibility of nurturing and giving took over their ability to care for themselves.

It is often during the stage when we are balancing family, work, and home responsibilities—or any combination of these— that there is a disconnection between ourselves and our health maintenance. How many times have you heard women say they have no time for themselves? As we work through seven simple steps to a healthier you, healthier living won't require more time; it will only require making better choices. I have been working for years to help women see the difference. And it is a huge difference.

Let's continue our evaluation by understanding how we can gain support for this venture toward wholeness, goodness, and strength. Your number one advocate should not be your best friend, your spouse, your children, or your personal trainer—it should be *you*. Unequivocally *you*. With a retraining of your mind and heart, you will be the first one to notice your strengths and weaknesses thoroughly. You will be the first in line at the supermarket with a cart full of nutritious food. And you will be the first to identify danger zone areas and people that have been a part of your unhealthy patterns for years—maybe decades.

The difficult part of evaluating ourselves is that we have been faithful to the bad habits and stumbling blocks in our lives. As unhealthy or unstable as these pitfalls might be, they still provide us with the comfort of what is known and familiar. Even an adventurous, outgoing, confident woman can be a creature of comfort and gravitate toward choices and behaviors that fit an unhealthy belief system she established long ago— even if it does not work in the slightest to her advantage.

We can overcome danger zone areas by having backup plans. Once we make a conscious decision to turn our lifestyles in a new direction, our heart, mind, and eyes will become aware of old patterns and habits that did not serve us well. We all have them. Again, the key is to identify those areas of weakness for you.

For example, a problem area for me is the gas station. Sounds funny, doesn't it? But I had developed a habit of purchasing a hot cappuccino from the machine every time I went into the gas station to pay for my gas. As a frugal person, I wanted to get the best deal for my money, so I purchased the largest size. They tasted so good that soon I found myself pulling into the gas station just for a cappuccino to warm me up during the winter months, even when I didn't need gas. It wasn't long before my pants were tight around the waist.

Next to your listed danger zone areas, write a solution you know you can achieve. Do not simply say "No longer buy such and such" or "No longer do such and such." Your plan of action needs to have specific steps. The more precise your backup plan is, the more you increase your chances of success.

Example:

Danger Zone Area	Problem	Solutions: Plan A/Plan B/Plan C/etc.
Gas station	Drinking cappuccinos often	Plan A: Buy hot flavored mint tea instead and sweeten with a sugar-free sweetener.
		Plan B: Pay for gas at pump and don't go into gas station.
		Plan C: Ask someone else in the car to go into the gas station to pay for the gas.
		Plan D: Ask spouse to fill up tank.
		Plan E: Go to different gas station that doesn't have the cappuccino machine.

When I try to refrain from buying movie theater popcorn, I go nuts during the movie smelling it, thinking about the popcorn, and hearing others munch on it so much that I cannot enjoy the movie.

Danger Zone Place	Problem	Solutions: Plan A/Plan B/ Plan C/etc.
Movie theater	Snacks	Plan A: Bring my own fat-free popcorn.
		Plan B: Avoid the movie theater altogether and rent a movie to watch at home.
		Plan C: Save enough fats, carbohydrates, and calories in my daily food intake to be able to eat it without guilt or shame.
		Plan D: Only go to the movies on a predetermined "free" day of eating without worrying.

Writing down an escape plan from cappuccinos and movie popcorn might not initially seem like a "simple step," but it is. Recognizing what has *not* worked in your daily routine is the only way to head toward real change. I would go as far as to say that if you have ever tried even one diet that did not work for you, then this is exactly the way to begin. The more backup plans we have, the better our chances for success are, and the more at ease our minds can be throughout the process.

The true purpose of these alternate plans for our choices is not to create a mind-boggling list of rules. The purpose is to deliberately change our behavior in the first few weeks so that we do not feel cornered by old habits but rather feel we have plenty of options. A diet is restrictive. A lifestyle change opens up possibilities. That is the difference that will make a difference in our results.

Use this chart for yourself. Use your journal if you need more help.

Danger Zone Places	Problem	Solutions: Plan A/Plan B/ Plan C
1.		Plan A:
		Plan B:
		Plan C:
2.		Plan A:
		Plan B:
		Plan C:
3.		Plan A:
		Plan B:
		Plan C:
4.		Plan A:
		Plan B:
		Plan C:
5.		Plan A:

		Plan B:
		Plan C:

Once you recognize danger zone areas or situations, you might stumble across a few surprise obstacles to health—people. Danger zone people. Actually, the danger is more about how *you* feel when around them than it is about the people themselves. The key is to recognize that certain people trigger your desire to eat. Acknowledge this so you can make a plan. Later, you might want to analyze the "why" further. But for now your simple goal is to write backup plans so you can survive the folks who bring out your inner eater.

When I was younger the very first thing I would do upon arriving at my in-laws was accept their offer of something sweet to eat. They were very hospitable, and my mother-in-law always had a generous supply of tantalizing treats—everything from sweet rolls to cookies to chocolates.

I hadn't even realized how hooked I was on eating her sweets until I went on a diet and noticed how stressful it was for me to visit their home without eating at the same time. We had always intertwined visiting with eating. Later on, when I took our daughters to visit her and she didn't have sweets, I was dismayed. What? No treats? Surely she had something in the freezer? What about her secret stash?

Alcoholics Anonymous encourages recovering alcoholics to stay away from what they call "wet faces and wet places." (The word "wet" refers to people or places with alcohol.) This is good advice for all of us who face temptations of any kind. Now, just getting healthy doesn't mean we have to avoid people—after all, there is much we love about the support of friends and family.

But we do need to look at the way we interact with certain folks.

You might have some friends who always seem to gather over food. Such gatherings are fun and an important part of life, but what if every now and then you introduced an alternate activity? Such as going for a long walk or heading to the bowling alley? Check your local entertainment listings and attend a lecture at the library or catch a performance by a music group. Even if food is involved at some point, at least you will be active as well. And now those friends will not always be your excuse to just sit and eat. They will be your reason to get out, interact, and experience new things.

Danger Zone People	Problem	Solutions: Plan A/Plan B/Plan C/etc.
My in-laws	Sweets	Plan A: When I go to visit them have gum or low-calorie mints with me.
		Plan B: Visit them on the phone instead.
		Plan C: Visit at mealtime, and bring a healthy dish with me.
		Plan D: Ask to visit in the living room instead of around the kitchen table.
		Plan E: Have a sugar-free drink to sip on.

Fill out your own chart. If needed use a journal for more writing space.

Danger Zone People	Problem	Solutions: Plan A/Plan B/ Plan C
1.		Plan A:
		Plan B:
		Plan C:
2.		Plan A:
		Plan B:
		Plan C:
3.		Plan A:
		Plan B:
		Plan C:
4.		Plan A:
		Plan B:
		Plan C:
5.		Plan A:
		Plan B:
		Plan C:

Support from Others

We are fortunate to have lots of choices when it comes to support when we want to make a change. However, the many options of diet programs, books, videos, and groups can cause us to fall back on the decision by indecision choice once again. Have you tried "every diet under the sun"? I have. Or at least I feel as though I have. Have you invested lots of money and time and effort into many different styles of healthy living? I have. After a few weeks of initial success and then eventual failure, I would write off the new diet as "not for me" or "not effective." But honestly, the problem with most of the diets was that I was not yet ready to commit or the method included elements that did not suit my life for one reason or another.

We are unique individuals, and God has a plan that will work best for you. The key to success is tapping into that source. I encourage you to go through the process of evaluating a few of your past methods so that you can figure out what *will* work for you as we go through the rest of the steps.

The following is an example of my evaluation of a few programs I have tried. I list the pros and cons for me personally.

Weight Watchers

Pros:

Support group meets regularly, teaches overall nutrition, portion sizes, encourages exercise, has helpful material and flexible eating plans, and offers accountability.

Cons:

Sometimes I became obsessed with the points system, though they now have a plan that doesn't require counting. There is an out-of-pocket fee, which helps initially with motivation but after a while also became difficult for us to manage in our budget.

Body for Life

Pros:

Excellent eating plan allowing freedom of choice, eating up to six times a day small, healthy serving sizes (the size of your fist of healthy carbohydrates and lean proteins the size of your palm). Support available free on phone 24 hours a day, seven days a week. Teaches overall nutrition, portion sizes, and flexible eating plans. Exercise is a must. Has helpful material on an inspirational level with before and after photos, has an incentive competition with big-dollar prizes, and recognition given to those who complete 12 weeks of their program.

Cons:

The weight training portion encourages you to go for "tens" on a scale of one to ten. The problem is if someone is not well trained, they can lift too much or lift improperly and actually cause injury to themselves. I was thrilled with my results; however, after the 12 weeks my joints were so sore I thought I had arthritis. My doctor told me I had been overtraining. Also the supplements that are recommended can be costly.

TOPS: Take Off Pounds Sensibly

Pros:

Support group meets regularly, focuses on the entire person (physically and spiritually), teaches how to have a healthy lifestyle, and offers accountability.

Cons:

Some of the meetings I went to felt more social in nature. And at the time I really needed a focused group of people for accountability, but with the right mix of people attending, I think it could have been a good match.

As you make your choice, take into consideration the types of food you like to eat and the type of exercise you either like to do or are willing to do in order for you to achieve optimum health for yourself. My personal list of attempted or considered plans goes on and on. But even from just these three personal reviews, I can see that two things I want in a program are accountability and reasonable cost.

I encourage you to talk to your friends, review your past efforts, and create the lists of pros and cons for a few programs. Then determine what your biggest needs are to feel comfortable with a program and, most importantly, to be able to stick with it.

Program Evaluation

Program or plan name:

Pros:

Cons:

Program or plan name:

Pros:

Cons:

Program or plan name:

Pros:

Cons:

Complete the following statements and use this information to fill out the Step One page of the Personal Plan for a Healthier Me in the back of this book: From my review of programs I have tried or that I have researched, I know that I need ___ _____ and _____ and _____ _____ from a plan. What does not work for me in a program is if that method is _____ and/or _____.

What It Takes

Already we have some significant tools for success—ways to identify our strengths and weaknesses and written plans of action to overcome danger zone places and faces.

The support you seek to make this time different can come in many different forms—a neighbor, a study group, an exercise class, a counselor, an online chat room, or a paid program. Possibly your support system will be a combination of several of these. And as we progress through the remaining simple steps to a healthier you, you will discover what that support could or should look like for your personal plan to be successful.

After thinking through your danger zone places and people, I encourage you to also assess those people and places that encourage healthy decisions and behaviors. If there is a coffee shop you can meet friends at instead of a doughnut shop, that might be a good choice for you. There are probably friends who play tennis on the weekends or go for walks every morning— find time to participate in these activities with them. There are positive choices everywhere you turn.

Choose people who are walking the walk and not just talking the talk. People who can share their experience, strength, and hope in order to encourage and inspire you. Don't choose someone or a group that has good intentions but doesn't follow through on their commitment. We all have a friend or two like that. They mean well, but they simply aren't truly committed to giving themselves the gift of being healthy. They frequently back out or don't follow through in joining you with your planned exercise together, or they set themselves up for failure.

Now that you are seriously making changes, you need someone you can count on, a role model, someone who can understand what you are going through. You need someone who will pat you on the back for a job well done and give you a helping hand up when you have fallen.

I would pray about it. This is not a light decision. Right off the top of your head you may know exactly who you want to ask, or you may have to pray about it for a while. You may live in such an unhealthy atmosphere that in your realm of friends and family you do not have a person who would qualify. In this case join a health club and tell the staff exactly what you are looking for. The more specific you can be, the greater your chances for success are in getting the kind of person you need.

Often health club employees are more than happy to be your accountability partners. I worked in health clubs for years, and my fellow employees and I were honored and flattered when someone asked for our help. As the sponsor or accountability partner of someone just starting a healthier lifestyle program, we also help ourselves in achieving our goals. It is one of those life truths: What you give out to others comes back to you.

In order to become the healthy person we know God wants us to be, we have got to be willing to let go of negative thoughts, feelings, attitudes, and behaviors that hinder our growth. Take time to be still. Go to God and ask Him to show you areas in your life that are hurting your process. Also seek to better understand your strengths so that when you seek support from people or programs, you will discover a good match.

The Satisfied Life

Connecting with others and finding ways to support your new healthy lifestyle will bring great satisfaction to your soul. What feels good already about the changes you are making and planning to make? Facing a life of satisfaction requires us to evaluate what does not satisfy us. Are you doing anything halfheartedly? Do you work or tend to other responsibilities with the frown of dissatisfaction? Allow the lessons you learn in the area of health and fitness to impact other areas of life.

Devotional Health

Either in this book or in your journal, write down the insights you have gained about your strengths and weaknesses. In what ways did you receive support in the past? In what ways did you not have support in the past? How will this time be different?

Prayer

God, help me discover the me You created me to be. May I seek Your strength as my foundation for all my efforts. May I also serve Your purpose for my life as I gain new understanding of what support looks like from people, places, and the process. Amen.

*Complete the Step One page
of your Personal Plan for a Healthier Me
at the back of the book.*

Step 2 | Create a New Relationship with Food

Most everyone in the health field or even on the street agrees vegetables get an A plus, and unless you are a vegetarian, most everyone agrees lean proteins, such as fish, chicken, turkey, and lean cuts of beef and pork, are part of a balanced diet. Both the American Heart and Diabetic Associations agree moderate amounts of low-fat dairy products are good for you, as well as fruits and whole grains.

Eating or drinking more than a little of processed carbohydrates without protein makes us crave more food. I look back at my food journals from years ago and am surprised how unhealthily I ate back then.

Example:

8:00 AM: 1 low-fat Pop-Tart or a bowl of low-fat (high-sugar) cereal with fat-free milk

10:00 AM: 2 handfuls low-fat potato chips, diet pop

Noon: 2 slices turkey lunchmeat on white bread sandwich, salad of lettuce and carrots with fat-free French salad dressing, 3 bites cheesecake, apple juice

2:00 PM: 3 reduced-fat cookies

3:00 PM: fat-free pretzels and caramel corn rice cakes, diet pop (I was hoping not to eat until dinner, but I am so hungry right now I have to eat something.)

5:00 PM: grilled chicken breast, fat-free mashed potatoes, reduced-fat roll with no butter (jelly instead), salad with fat-free dressing, diet pop

7:00 PM: fat-free frozen yogurt and diet pop

Sure I was eating low fat, yet I struggled to keep my caloric intake low enough to stay at the *high end* of my ideal body weight, even though I taught aerobic exercise classes. I was always preoccupied with what I could eat and when. I was a prisoner of my own appetite and was in the emotionally frustrating bondages that the chains of usually craving something more to eat, especially craving sweets, held me. I hated it. I barely ever felt satisfied.

All those fat-free, highly processed products were loaded with sugars. Here I thought I was being good because I was staying away from candy. Yet all those snacks, white breads, and highly processed foods digest in our bodies a lot like white sugar. No wonder I was craving sweets. My body was on carbohydrate overload, and I never knew it.

Study after study reports eating a low-fat lifestyle is very helpful in obtaining and maintaining good health physically. The majority of Americans who are in hospitals today are in for the same reason—their lifestyle. Cancer, heart disease, diabetes, and high blood pressure all thrive on a high-fat diet.

The word "diet" in today's society has almost become a curse word. "Diet" does not mean starvation or depravation. Whatever each of us consumes through food and beverages is our daily diet.

Unfortunately, as low fat became more available people began thinking they no longer had to be concerned with portion size. This misconception could not be further from the truth. Thus, Americans (especially) have become more overweight as a society than ever before.

When it comes to eating, I think the key to becoming healthy and maintaining good health for busy people is to create a diet of nutritious foods that are low in fat and high in fiber, that have a low number of calories per serving, and taste good.

One thing we know for sure, fat is higher in condensed calories at a whopping nine calories per gram compared to carbohydrates and lean proteins, which are both four calories per gram, and alcohol, which is seven calories per gram. We can eat two and a quarter more grams of lean proteins and carbohydrates than fats for the same amount of calories. Calorie for calorie, you are getting more bang for your caloric buck when you eat low fat vs. high fat.

What foods are holding you back?

What are some high-fat foods that are hard for you to stop eating?

What are some foods you know you cannot have in the house without them screaming for you to eat them?

Let's first look at how you have treated food in the past. Finish these observations with the appropriate word(s) and then complete the closing statement.

I have treated food as though its purpose is _____

_____.

Food became a source of _____ and

_____.

The only time I had a happy relationship with food was

_____.

I was the most anxious about food when _____

_____.

During the day, I thought about food _____

_____.

I would justify overeating or depriving myself because ____

_____.

My relationship with food was tied to the following emotions _____

_____.

I have treated food as if it didn't have value. I have treated food the way I treat _____.

My new attitude toward food will include _____

_____.

Often overweight people don't necessarily eat a large quantity of food, but they are eating a lot of what I called compact or condensed calorie foods that rob them from achieving their goals.

When I was facilitating weight loss and healthier living classes, I regularly met with frustrated people who were eating little and yet were unable to lose weight and were hungry all the time. Some were even gaining weight.

How can this be? It is simple—condensed calories, which are foods that are loaded with a lot of calories for a very little portion size, sabotage our weight loss efforts and weight maintenance goals. Simple examples are potato chips at a whopping 150 calories for about a handful, nuts (even though they are healthy, they are very high in calories), and peanut butter (180 calories for two tiny tablespoons).

Think of calories as money. Each calorie represents one dollar. You have so many calories to spend a day, depending on your goals. Keeping track of calories as you would money is a safe bet, especially if you are a bargain shopper like me. Don't you just love finding a super deal on something you wanted? That's the way it can be with eating too, if you learn how to shop using your calorie dollars wisely. There is no special formula; you don't have to count points or anything like that. You simply want to choose food and beverages that give you a lot of delicious, tasty, satisfying options for as few calories as possible.

With gas prices being as high as they are, aren't you happy to get more for your money when prices are low and you can fill up your automobile tank for a fraction of the cost it takes to fill it up when prices are high? That's the way it is with bargain eating. We want to get as much as we can to feel satisfied with as few caloric dollars as possible.

If you are an average woman, consuming 1200 to 1400 calories per day is a good weight loss goal. So you have 1200 to 1400 calorie dollars a day to spend. You don't want to consume less than this because you could lower your metabolic rate. Quite the reverse is desired; we want to increase our basal metabolic rate so we will naturally burn off more calories through the day without even trying. (Exercise will increase your basal metabolic rate, and we'll talk about workout options in Step Four.) We want to eat foods that are relatively lower in caloric dollars than some of their counterparts.

For example, fat-free Italian salad dressing is a great value with only 12 calorie dollars for two tablespoons vs. high-fat Italian salad dressing at an expensive 140 calorie dollars for the same quantity. This simple change saves you 128 calorie dollars. If you ate the higher calorie option, you would need to take an extra mile-and-a-quarter walk. That is a pretty high price to pay, don't you agree? And that is just for salad, which should be one of the lowest-calorie foods we can eat.

Below are some examples of how to "shop" wisely with your caloric dollars. The first food listed is the one with compacted calories and the second food is a healthier, lighter choice. Notice the many calories saved simply by making some minor substitutions.

> 1 piece blueberry pie (650 calories) traded for 2 cups
> blueberries in sugar-free blueberry pie glaze and 2

tablespoons fat-free whipped topping (138 calories) = caloric dollars saved: $512

½ cup premium ice cream (150 calories) traded for ½ cup fat-free frozen yogurt (50 calories) = caloric dollars saved: $100

1 tablespoon mayonnaise (110 calories) traded for light mayonnaise (30 calories) = caloric dollars saved: $80

1 cup potato salad (300 calories) traded for 1 cup new potatoes (120 calories) = caloric dollars saved: $180

1 cup pineapple in heavy syrup (216 calories) traded for 1 cup fresh pineapple (76 calories) = caloric dollars saved: $140

1 biscuit (4½ ounce) with 1 tablespoon butter (570 calories) traded for 1 slice light toast with 1 tablespoon fruit spread (75 calories) = caloric dollars saved: $495

1 cup granola cereal (400 calories) traded for 1 cup Wheaties cereal (110 calories) = caloric dollars saved: $290

1 bagel (400 calories) traded for 2 slices light toast (80 calories) = caloric dollars saved: $320

2 toaster pastries (420 calories) traded for 2 low-fat waffles with sugar-free syrup (140 calories) = caloric dollars saved: $280

1 ounce cheese curls (150 calories) traded for 1 ounce cheese-flavored rice cakes (60 calories) = caloric dollars saved: $90

3 ounces ground beef hamburger (260 calories) traded for

3 ounces ground eye of round (141 calories) = caloric dollars saved: $119

4 ounces fried shrimp (274 calories) traded for 4 ounces boiled shrimp (112 calories) = caloric dollars saved: $162

2 tablespoons Italian salad dressing (140 calories) traded for 2 tablespoons fat-free Italian salad dressing (12 calories) = caloric dollars saved: $128

1 tablespoon real butter (100 calories) traded for 1 tablespoon half-fat butter (50 calories) = caloric dollars saved: $50

3 cups butter-flavored popcorn (210 calories) traded for 3 cups light popcorn (70 calories) = caloric dollars saved: $140

1 Snickers candy bar (278 calories) traded for a York Peppermint Patty (180 calories) = caloric dollars saved: $98

Grand total of high-fat, unhealthy choices: **4628 calories**

Grand total of low-fat, healthier choices: **1444 calories**

Simply by making minor changes, we saved 3184 calories, just shy of the 3500 calories we need to burn to lose a pound.

These are perfect examples that little changes make a big difference. Beware of the foods and beverages listed below that are calorie dense:

pie crust

nuts

fried foods

cream base soups

sodas (not sugar free)

fatty cuts of meat, such as cheap hamburger

hot dogs

salami

high-fat ice creams

sugary syrups

chocolate

oils

fats

regular salad dressings

mayonnaise

regular Miracle Whip

half-and-half

whipping cream

regular sour cream

butter

margarine

fruit juices

granola

cookies

candy

frosting

pastries

potato chips

most processed snack
    foods

fatty lunch meats

all regular cheeses

avocados

One thing I strongly discourage people from doing is drinking their calories. A quick drink of a small glass of orange juice is almost double the calories of eating a small orange or two small tangerines. Eating is more time consuming and satisfying. Save your calories for food; don't spend them on drinks.

An enlightening exercise is to take a look at a nutrition book, which should have calories, fat, protein, and other information for individual foods broken down. If you don't have one of these books, go get one soon. I'll bet even your local used bookstore has some on hand. Take some time to go through the book with a marker and highlight the food choices you enjoy eating that are lower in calories and also low in fat.

When you run across a food you have been eating or that you love but that is high in calories and fat, write that one down on a separate sheet or underline it in the book. This is a good reminder of the foods you will need to be the most aware of.

Now make a written list of your favorite things you have highlighted. Keep this list with you or have copies in convenient places such as the kitchen and in your car, so that you are able to easily make healthier food choices. The goal is for these choices to become automatic.

Sometimes all it takes to be your ideal weight is a little knowledge and some small changes in what you eat. I can't tell you how many of my students throughout the years have thought they knew a lot about foods. They felt they didn't need to go through a calorie-counting book and highlight lower calorie food choices as I had suggested. But in my office the following week, sitting there with their food journal and feeling proud of the changes they had made in their eating (thinking they had made healthier, lower-caloric food choices), they were often disappointed and sometimes had even gained weight. Why? Because they switched to foods they thought were lower in calories but actually were more calorie dense.

Does eating healthier, lower-fat foods mean you will never eat any high-calorie foods again? Most likely not; however, these foods will be eaten when you make a conscious choice to wander from your day in, day out eating plan. Eating high-calorie foods will not be the norm any longer because you will want to enjoy as much quantity of quality food as you can for your caloric dollars so that you will feel satisfied.

Often, when you decide to make the switch to eating lower-calorie foods, you will become satisfied without completely eating all that is on your plate.

The Satisfied Life

Meals or dining experiences are often described as "satisfying." We delight in filling up, easing our hunger, and tasting a variety of flavors. While eating is a necessity, it is also a pleasure. A satisfied life will include savoring simple pleasures. And a healthy life will include discovering pleasure beyond those on the plate. Consider what gives you joy. Is it a conversation with a good friend? Going to a romantic comedy? Walking alongside a rushing river? Sitting in the sun with a good book and a glass of iced tea? Seek the satisfied life.

Devotional Health

Spend a day allowing yourself to be still before you eat. Don't rush into a meal; instead, spend just a few minutes in prayer. Enjoy your meal and then be still again. How do you feel after a few minutes of eating? Are you full, satisfied?

Give thanks for the gift of food and health. Let your heart be full and satisfied as well as your stomach.

Prayer

Lord, fill my spirit and heart with gratitude today. Ease my hunger for attention or acceptance in the world with Your unconditional love. May I live each day as a valued, vital stretch of time so that I live a life of fulfillment and purpose. Amen.

*Complete the Step Two page
of your Personal Plan for a Healthier Me
at the back of the book.*

Doing Things Light

- Make the preparation of your meal part of the pleasure experience.

- Leave space on your plate—fight the urge to fill it.

- Drink a glass of water after eating and wait ten minutes before considering seconds.

- Include three different colors on your plate, incorporating vegetables, grains, and protein.

- Enjoy eating. Savor each bite and appreciate the flavors.

- Start with a salad or a bowl of soup if you are always hungry after a meal.

- Serve yourself the appropriate size serving of protein (size of your palm) and carbohydrates (size of your fist), and if you are still hungry, eat only green vegetables.

- Eat at the table in a relaxed atmosphere.

Step 3 | Practice Intentional Eating

You might worry that by focusing on what you eat and giving food careful consideration, you could become obsessed with it. But I can tell you from experience that when you switch to a mind-set of eating intentionally and for the purpose of energy, health, and pleasure, you will find that you are freed from the bondage that comes with frequent dieting.

Even just five years ago I would not have believed that this shift could happen. Ever since those days in school when I was worried about my weight, I have been determined to use food as a reward/punishment system. The only value I assigned to what I was eating was whether or not it would make me fat. But even when I was worried about my weight, it came not from a desire for health but from the need for validation and approval from others. If someone had said to me, "We have a pill that will take away your appetite and cravings for three months straight. You'll never want to eat again," I would have stood there with my hand out, eager to get that pill and be unconcerned about my body's need for fuel. That's how unhealthy my thinking was.

In this chapter we will look at ways to change our eating patterns and, more importantly, change our thinking patterns about eating and living. We will acknowledge that food is a necessity and a pleasure in our lives and that it is also key to longevity and vitality.

Of all the programs I have seen or experienced, the simplest ones seem to offer the most success. They blend a healthy lifestyle that encompasses all kinds of priorities. The ones that require complicated methods or systems often take over a person's life. They don't produce permanent change, but rather stir up an obsessive mind-set we can all experience at one time or another.

What You Need

In order to know what we need, we need to know what our body spends when it is at its ideal healthy weight. This information is called our basal metabolic rate (BMR). Achieving and maintaining our healthy weight is our goal.

The following formula will tell you how many calories you need per day to maintain a certain weight. Write your answers for each step on the line provided.

1. Multiply the goal weight you want to be in pounds by 4.4 and then add 655 = Answer A _____

2. Multiply your height in inches by 4.3 = Answer B _____

3. Multiply your age in years by 4.7 = Answer C _____

4. Add (A) _____ with (B) _____ and subtract (C) _____
   = (your resting BMR)

5. Take your basal metabolic rate number and multiply it by the activity factor number that best describes your lifestyle below. This number is the number of calories you need to maintain the healthy weight you want.

   1.2 for sedentary lifestyle

   1.4 for moderately active life style

   1.6 for vigorously active lifestyle

Example: A 5' 7" (67 inches tall) female who is 43 years old and has a sedentary lifestyle feels best having her ideal healthy weight at 145 pounds. Using these facts with the formula provided lets figure her BMR.

1. 145 pounds x 4.4 + 655 = 1293

2. 67 x 4.3 = 288.1 (drop any number after the decimal = 288)

3. 43 x 4.7 = 202.1 (drop any number after the decimal = 202)

4. 1293 + 288 - 202 = 1379

5. 1379 x 1.2 = 1654.8 (drop any number after the decimal = 1654)

   Answer: This woman only needs 1654 calories per day to maintain her ideal healthy weight.

Figure your BMR and record it in your Personal Plan for a Healthier Me at the end of the book.

The K.I.S.S. of Success

The acronym in the K.I.S.S. eating plan stands for "Keep It Smart and Simple" because that is what busy women need. You can use your choice of support systems or programs and still incorporate the K.I.S.S. sensibility. Your earlier evaluation of what you need in a program or health routine will help you know what to include, rule out, and embrace as we discuss this plan.

I will present seven simple breakfast menus, seven simple lunch menus, and seven simple dinner menus along with a long list of snacks that you can have up to three times a day. If you are not hungry you can skip the snacks. Breakfast, lunch, and dinners should always be eaten to maintain healthy sugar levels in the bloodstream and reduce mood swings and fatigue. You should also get the recommended seven to eight hours of sleep daily along with this eating plan. When you are tempted to bypass lunch because you are busy, remember that skipping meals will slow down the body's metabolism.

To simplify the K.I.S.S. plan we'll use your tightly clenched fist as a gauge of the serving size for carbohydrates and the size of your palm (without the fingers) for proteins. The only time we'll include the fingers in our serving size of proteins is when we eat broiled, steamed, poached, or grilled fish with no added fat. What's nice about using this form of measuring is that a large man will have a larger serving size than that of a petite woman, making our portion sizes appropriate for the size of person we are.

This fist and palm method of measuring is a rough gauge, and when trying to decide whether to have a little smaller or tad bit larger serving size of any food, select the smaller portion size. If you feel comfortable or full before that serving is totally eaten, stop eating. Cover and save the food in the refrigerator as a snack for later.

Eating little quantities throughout the day just until you feel full or satisfied is known as grazing. Grazing on healthy, low-fat foods helps keep the chemistry of our blood sugar levels in a healthy range to reduce highs and lows in our energy levels throughout the day. The key is grazing small amounts of lower calorie, healthier food choices throughout the day and not gorging in any one meal.

The meal options are interchangeable, so you can have confidence in knowing you will always be staying within 1400 calories or less per day. In order for a meal to be considered for the K.I.S.S. plan, it had to be easy to prepare using easy-to-find grocery store ingredients; be nutritious, delicious, and satisfying; and easy to clean up as well. Tell me, could it get any easier than this?

For each meal, choose one of the seven options. A simple way to plan would be to use the first of each meal offerings for day one, the second of each meal offerings for day two, and continue from there so that you would not repeat any of the meals in a full week. However, if you are like me, you will end up finding some favorites that you want to have regularly. I encourage you to try the first week as a variety sampler.

K.I.S.S. Meal Plan Breakfasts

French Toast

    Prepare with light bread, egg whites, and skim milk. Spritz toast with fat-free margarine spray and top with sugar-free maple syrup

    Low-carb milk

    Coffee or tea

Hot Cereal

Prepare 1 serving (which is about 1 cup for women) Cream of Wheat or real oatmeal as directed on box with water and Splenda as sweetener and/or sugar-free maple syrup.

Low-carb milk

Coffee or tea

Breakfast Sandwich or Breakfast Roll Up

Prepare using light bread toast or fat-free soft tortillas, 2 egg whites or ¼ cup egg substitute, 1 tablespoon real bacon bits or 1 slice Canadian bacon, and 1 slice fat-free American, Cheddar, or Swiss cheese, if desired. For 1 minute (or until fully cooked), cook the eggs in a microwave-safe bowl that has been sprayed with nonfat cooking spray. The egg will puff up as it cooks and deflate as it cools. If using bacon, stir the bacon bits in with the egg before cooking. While the egg is cooking, put your bread in the toaster. Place cooked egg on toast. If using Canadian bacon, cook it for 5 seconds in the microwave, just enough to heat it. Place Canadian bacon on top of egg. Place cheese on top of hot cooked egg and top with second piece of toast. Cover with towel for a minute to let the heat from the egg melt the cheese. If desired, season with light salt, pepper, Tabasco sauce, mustard, or ketchup.

Coffee or tea

Breakfast Scrambles

Prepare in a nonstick skillet coated lightly with nonfat cooking spray. Cook a fist-sized portion of your favorite vegetables until tender. Consider trying tomatoes, onions, broccoli, turnip greens, chives, spinach, squash, zucchini, or mushrooms. Add ½ cup egg substitute with 1 tablespoon real bacon bits, 1 slice Canadian bacon, or lean ham, chopped. Stir constantly until egg is fully cooked. If desired, season with light salt, pepper, Tabasco sauce, mustard, or ketchup.

1 slice light bread, toasted, with sugar-free fruit spread

1 of either: ½ orange, ½ grapefruit, or other citrus-based fruit the size of your fist

Coffee or tea

Scrambled Eggs

Combine ½ cup egg substitute or 4 egg whites (with yellow food coloring added if desired) with 1 tablespoon skim milk. Season with light salt and pepper to taste and cook in a nonstick skillet that has been sprayed with nonfat cooking spray.

1 of either: ½ orange, ½ grapefruit, or other citrus-based fruit the size of your fist

1 slice light bread, toasted, with sugar-free fruit spread

Coffee or tea

Pancakes

Create a short stack of pancakes about the size of your fist using reduced-fat pancake mix (make as directed on box with water) in a nonstick skillet sprayed with nonfat cooking spray.

Choice of: 2 vegetarian sausage links or 2 slices Canadian bacon

Sugar-free maple syrup

Coffee or tea

*C*old Cereal

Any cold cereal with no added sugar that is approximately 100 calories or less for a 1-cup serving (examples: Wheaties, Total, Special K)

1 cup low-carb milk

Noncaloric sweetener, such as Splenda

Coffee or tea

K.I.S.S. Meal Plan Lunches

*S*andwiches or Mini Hoagies with a Fresh Vegetable Tray

Choose from one of the following lunch meats a portion the size of your palm:* lean roast beef, lean ham, lean honey ham, lean maple-flavored ham, turkey, smoked turkey, or chicken. Place on light bread, toasted or plain. Use fat-free hamburger buns or fat-free hot dog buns for hoagies. Top with any of the following: light Miracle Whip or light mayonnaise, fat-free salad dressing, mustard, ketchup, lettuce, tomato, onion, and one large dill pickle on the side.

Side dish: Prepare fresh cucumber slices, red bell pepper slices, green bell pepper slices, yellow bell pepper slices, orange bell pepper slices, fresh broccoli florets, or celery sticks as you'd like with up to 2 tablespoons fat-free salad dressing for dipping.

*G*arden Salad with Protein

Slice up cucumbers, onions, radishes, green pepper, broccoli, cherry tomatoes, mushrooms, and up to 2 tablespoons fat-free

---

* Keep in mind that the palm portion does not include fingers.

salad dressing on top of 5 ounces of fresh garden green lettuce. Top salad with a palm portion of one of the following meats: lean roast beef, lean ham, turkey, smoked turkey, or chicken.

Turn this into a chicken Caesar salad by using 2 tablespoons fat-free Caesar salad dressing and a palm portion of grilled or broiled chicken breast cut into thin strips.

Tuna or Chicken Salad Sandwiches or Salads

Combine 1 (6-ounce) can tuna in water or 98 percent fat-free chicken breast with 1 tablespoon fat-free Miracle Whip or fat-free salad dressing and 2 tablespoons light Miracle Whip or light mayonnaise, 1 stalk finely chopped celery, and 1 teaspoon sweet relish. For sandwiches, spread on light bread and top with lettuce. For salads, put a palm-portion size of the mixture on a bowl of your favorite fresh salad greens. You can use up to 2 tablespoons fat-free salad dressing for your greens as well.

Fresh Fruit Bowl

Take ½ of either a fresh cantaloupe or honeydew melon, remove the seeds, and place a fist-sized portion of cottage cheese into the hollowed-out center of the melon. Cut off the bottom of the outside of the melon to make it flat so the melon will sit like a bowl. If fresh melon isn't in season or available, have a fist-sized portion of canned tropical fruit salad in light syrup or light fruit cocktail with ½ cup fat-free cottage cheese.

Soup's On

1 cup of any low-fat soup with 5 low-fat crackers and 1 slice fat-free American or fat-free Cheddar cheese. Have along with an assortment of vegetables or a green salad with 2 tablespoons fat-free dressing.

Grilled Cheese Sandwich

Coat one side each of 2 slices light bread with ½ tablespoon of half-fat butter (not margarine) and place 2 slices of either fat-free Cheddar, fat-free Swiss, or fat-free American cheese in between the two slices of buttered bread and grill in a nonstick skillet until crispy golden brown on each side. Enjoy a large dill pickle on the side.

Side dish: Have as many fresh cucumber slices, red bell pepper slices, green bell pepper slices, yellow bell pepper slices, orange bell pepper slices, fresh broccoli florets, or celery sticks as you'd like with up to 2 tablespoons fat-free salad dressing for dipping.

OR

Grilled Ham and Cheese Sandwich

Prepare as above and add 2 slices lean ham on top of the cheese before you grill.

Side dish: Have as many fresh cucumber slices, red bell pepper slices, green bell pepper slices, yellow bell pepper slices, orange bell pepper slices, fresh broccoli florets, or celery sticks as you'd like with up to 2 tablespoons fat-free salad dressing for dipping.

Chinese Food

Enjoy 1 cup wonton soup or 1 cup Chinese vegetable soup or 1 cup hot-and-sour soup and 1½ cups of any stir-fry or steamed mixed vegetables with scallops, shrimp, beef, or chicken. Example: chicken and broccoli, shrimp and mixed vegetables, etc. Oh yes, and 1 fortune cookie (at only 30 calories). If you are dining at a Chinese restaurant, request no nuts, rice, egg roll, spring roll, and anything else they might add as a side dish.

K.I.S.S. Meal Plan Dinners

Once you make your dinner selection, you can add a tossed fresh garden salad made with your choice of the following: any kind of lettuce, sliced fresh tomatoes, carrots, radishes, and cucumbers with up to 2 tablespoons fat-free salad dressing.

Smothered Steak, Pork Tenderloin, or Chicken Dinner

Choose one palm-sized serving from any of the following: boneless, skinless chicken breast, pork tenderloin, or beef steaks (eye of round, top round steak, lean sirloin, tenderloin, flank steak (also known as London broil steak), chopped eye of round, or extra lean ground beef. Make sure all visible fat is removed before cooking.). A George Foreman or other similar grill works great for this dinner. For the best tasting steaks, cook on a high heat about two to three minutes per side with your favorite steak-seasoning blend. Do not add fat, butter, or oil to the skillet, grill, or broiler.

Prepare a fist-sized portion of mushrooms and onions per serving, sliced and cooked in a nonstick skillet with the lid on, in ½ tablespoon half-fat butter. Sprinkle lightly with garlic salt. Put the cooked onions-and-mushrooms mixture over each serving of meat.

Side dish: One choice of ½ ear of corn on the cob, a fist-sized baked potato, or a fist-sized baked sweet potato topped with no more than ½ tablespoon half-fat butter or fat-free sour cream or salsa. (To prepare either kind of potato, quickly pierce potatoes with a fork numerous times, wrap in a damp towel, and cook in the microwave for about 3 minutes. After 3 minutes, cook at 30-second intervals until fully cooked.

Pasta with Marinara Sauce

Take any form of cooked pasta, such as angel hair, spaghetti, rotini, shells, or ziti and top with a fist-sized serving of your favorite fat-free spaghetti sauce cooked with lean crumbled ground beef, low-fat crumbled turkey Italian sausage, or crumbled vegetarian beef or sausage. To substantially lower calories, substitute rinsed and squeeze-dried sauerkraut instead of pasta. It's quite tasty.

Seafood Lovers Delight Dinner

Have you ever heard the joke, "I'm on a seafood diet. Whenever I see food, I eat it." Okay, so the joke might not be so good, but this seafood dinner is a winner.

I like eating fish because one serving of any of the following fish grilled, steamed, or baked is the size of your entire hand. To steam or bake, put the fish on a piece of heavy-duty foil that has been sprayed with nonfat cooking spray, season with lemon-pepper seasoning, and fold the foil up like a package. Bake at 350 degrees for 15 to 20 minutes or until fully cooked, depending on thickness of the fish. Fish choices are: swordfish, orange roughy, whitefish, haddock, lobster, crab, or shrimp. Salmon is another good choice, but it has to be the size of your palm only.

Side dishes: A fist-sized serving of steamed brown or wild rice, or corn, squash, pasta, beans, baked sweet potato, or red skins. A fist-sized portion of cooked vegetables. Use butter-flavored sprinkles to flavor along with a little garlic salt.

Frittata

A frittata is a lot like an omelet but much easier to make. In a nonstick skillet that has been sprayed with nonfat cooking spray, cook a fist-sized portion of your favorite vegetables for a few minutes until tender. You can select any combination of vegetables your heart desires. Vegetable choices include but are not limited to: tomatoes, onions, broccoli, spinach, chives, zucchini, and/or mushrooms. Once tender, add ½ cup egg substitute with 1 tablespoon real bacon bits, 1 slice Canadian bacon, or chopped lean ham. Cook over medium heat until almost set. In the meantime preheat the oven. Once the frittata is fully cooked around the edges, place the entire skillet in the oven on the top rack and bake at 350 degrees until the frittata no longer wiggles in the center (approximately 5 minutes).

Garlic bread: Toast 1 slice of light bread (any flavor) and then spread ½ tablespoon half-fat butter on toast and lightly sprinkle it with garlic salt.

Side dish: Prepare low-fat coleslaw by mixing a 10-ounce bag of shredded coleslaw mix (cabbage, red cabbage, and carrots) with a ½ cup light coleslaw dressing mix. Or you can choose a fist-sized serving of any of the following cooked vegetables in any combination you'd like: broccoli, asparagus, cauliflower, green beans, spinach, zucchini, turnip greens, collard greens, or onion. Use butter-flavored sprinkles to flavor along with a little garlic salt.

Souper Easy Dinner

Two 1-cup servings of any low-fat or fat-free soup, stew, or chili in a clear or tomato based broth made with vegetables and lean meats. There are plenty premade fat-free and low-fat soups and chilies on the market today. My *Busy People's* cookbooks are loaded with fantastic fat-free and low-fat soup, stew, and chili recipes. Slow cookers are superb for these types of dinners. For a can't-fail recipe, put 1 48-ounce can of V-8 vegetable juice in a slow cooker with either 2 10-ounce cans of 98 percent fat-free chicken or canned beef and 2 1-pound bags of your favorite mixed vegetables. Cover and cook on low for 6 to 8 hours.

Special Family Roast Dinner

This is another wonderful recipe for your slow cooker. The secret is to select lean cuts of meat, such as eye of round beef roast, top sirloin roast, beef tenderloin roast, or even pork tenderloin roast. We can use extra lean roasts (with all visible fat removed) because the meat is tenderized as it cooks slowly. Plan on 4 ounces of raw meat per serving, which will cook down to a serving size about the size of a lady's palm. For every serving of meat, add a fist-sized serving of each of the following to the slow cooker: baby carrots, quartered onions, and, last but not least, peeled and cubed turnips, which will taste very much like potatoes when they are done cooking in this method. Stir a 1-ounce envelope of dry onion soup mix with 2 cups of water and pour over everything. Cover and cook on low for 8 to 9 hours.

Southwestern Fiesta Dinner

Use vegetarian meatless crumbles or extra lean ground beef or shredded chicken breast cooked with 1 envelope taco seasoning mix as directed on back of taco seasoning package. Sprinkle a palm-sized serving of cooked and seasoned taco meat over as much lettuce as you want. The lettuce will be your filler; however, you are not going to use more than 2 tablespoons of fat-free salad dressing, so don't use too much lettuce. Sprinkle the top of the seasoned meat and lettuce with the following combination of any of these ingredients you want, adding up to but not more than the size of your fist: fat-free shredded Cheddar cheese, fat-free or low-fat crushed tortilla chips, chopped tomato, fat-free sour cream, chopped onion, and chopped red or green bell pepper.

OR

Prepare taco-or fajita-seasoned extra lean beef or chicken breast the size of your palm. Add a fist-sized serving of grilled or steamed vegetables and a fist-sized serving of brown rice.

K.I.S.S. Meal Plan Snack List

You may have up to three snacks a day. Use your fist to measure portion size unless otherwise noted:

small apple

small orange

small pear

½ a small cantaloupe

½ small honeydew

½ small muskmelon

strawberries

blackberries

red raspberries

blueberries

watermelon

carrots with fat-free salad dressing as a dip

celery with low-fat or fat-free salad dressing as a dip

celery with fat-free cream cheese in the center (in moderation)

grape or cherry tomatoes

lean beef or turkey jerky (in moderation)

low-fat popcorn (3 fist-sized servings after it's popped)

low-fat or fat-free vegetable soup

fruit cups in pear juice

fat-free, no-sugar-added frozen yogurt

fat-free or low-fat cottage cheese

shrimp cocktail

extra lean lunch meats: turkey, ham, or roast beef thinly sliced and rolled (palm size)

sugar-free Popsicles

sugar-free, fat-free fudge bars

fat-free hot dog with light bread

fat-free potato chips or tortilla chips

K.I.S.S. Meal Plan Freebies

No need to worry about quantity, but still practice moderation:

celery

fresh mushrooms

green bell pepper

red bell pepper

yellow bell pepper

orange bell pepper

sugar-free gum, mints, sodas, and other beverages

cucumber slices in fat-free salad dressing

Below are the recommended servings for about 1400 to 1600 calories per day according to the USDA's new 2005 dietary guidelines:

fruits—4 servings

vegetables—3 to 4 servings

meat—2 3-ounce servings of low-fat fish, lean beef, lean pork, chicken breast, turkey breast,

tuna, egg substitute, egg whites

grains—6 servings

low-fat dairy—2 to 3 servings

fats/oils—2 tablespoons

Whenever possible avoid white sugar, white flour, fat, and processed foods. These will most likely be the items you will choose to occasionally splurge on, but remember to add the calories into your daily calorie count (figured on basal metabolic rate). Consider the following questions to help you evaluate your understanding of calories and your past consideration of them.

Have you ever written down exactly what you ate and added up the calories you consumed in a normal day?

Were you surprised? If so, why? What surprised you?

Are you aware of some unhealthy eating habits you have that you know you want to change?

Every successful weight-loss program or healthy eating program I have seen has had two things in common: The participants made a conscious effort to be aware of the foods they were eating, and most people documented what they ate. If you documented what you ate, would you eat with more awareness? Does the thought of being straightforward about what you eat and writing down on paper how much you eat scare you?

Sometimes we consume mass quantities of calories without even realizing it or enjoying it. I call this eating in the "Zoned-Out Zone." Sometimes we don't even realize we do it until it is too late and the bag of reduced-fat chips is gone. We had good intentions of eating only a few, but somehow between the first bite and the last crumb we became unaware of how much we were eating or even the fact that we were eating.

Focus on making progress, and don't get discouraged when you fall short of perfection. Record your answers here or in your journal.

Write down three positive eating changes you are going to make in your day today:

1.

2.

3.

Write down three things you are going to do today toward making your goal of being healthier a reality:

1.

2.

3.

Write down three things you ate that were very healthy today:

1.

2.

3.

Eating intentionally will change your approach toward eating and your attitude toward food.

The Satisfied Life

Discerning when you are full is a cultivated art. Sometimes we learn the hard way, by overindulging and feeling sick or feeling the pressure of our clothes tight against us. But the key to healthy eating is to stop before you reach the point of discomfort. And where we err in our eating practices, we often fail in just the opposite way in life practices. We stop ourselves from living fully too soon. We avoid risks, we step away from change, and we guard our hearts from expanding and feeling more deeply. As you learn to put the fork down before you get too full, consider how to dig deeper into your life. Give yourself permission to taste life's offerings of possibility and hope spoonful after spoonful.

Devotional Health

Take a prayer walk today as you decide upon your meal plan for the next few days or for the week. Ask for strength as you plan and for commitment as you face obstacles or past behaviors. If possible, take a prayer walk in addition to your planned exercise. As you put one step in front of the other, give yourself and your day over to God.

Prayer

God, help me be intentional in every aspect of my life. As I care for myself, my family, and those around me, may I rely on my faith in You to direct me toward intentional giving and living. I want to be a person who walks with the assurance that comes with purposed choices and decisions. Keep me healthy and mindful of what is right. Amen.

> *Complete the Step Three page of your Personal Plan for a Healthier Me at the back of the book.*

A Special Treat

Steamers: At night I like to make these with 1 percent or skim milk because the milk has medicinal properties that help the body relax and sleep better. Remember the olden days when someone couldn't sleep and Grandma would say, "Have a cup of hot milk with honey"? This is the same principle with a lot less fat and calories. During the day I like to make them with low-carb milk because it has more protein and less carbohydrates, which I feel gives me more energy. Here's the basic recipe. Feel free to be creative and make your own variations.

1   cup hot milk (heat in the microwave for 1 minute and 20 to 30 seconds)

2   tablespoons fat-free, low-carb liquid creamer— any flavor

2   to 3 individual serving size packets Splenda or other noncaloric sweetener

A few drops of your favorite flavoring or extract used for baking. Some of my favorites are vanilla, coconut, and almond.

Put all of the ingredients in blender and cover, but leave a slight crack between the lid and the blender for the heat to release. Pulse for about 30 seconds or until frothy. Pour into a mug. Drink hot.

Step **4** | **Move in the Right Direction**

One of the keys to success in your exercise program, whether you are just beginning or you are a lifetime athlete, might surprise you. It is something that many people love to do anyway—and that is sleep. A consistent exercise program that you'll stick with for the long haul begins by getting to bed in plenty of time so you can wake up well rested.

Try to get in the habit of exercising daily first thing in the morning. We often have good intentions to get our exercise done early in the day, but what happens when we get to bed late and decide to sleep in the extra half hour we originally planned to exercise? *I'll exercise after I get the children off to school.*

We get the kids off to school but then decide to start some laundry before work. *I'll exercise during my lunch hour.*

During our lunch hour we are busy with extra things the boss wanted done. *I'll exercise right after work.*

After work we remember we have a few errands to run before rushing home to start dinner. *I'll exercise right after dinner.*

After dinner we help the children with homework. *I'll exercise right after I get the children to bed.*

We get the children to bed and guess what? You know it. We are too tired. And with the best of intentions we think, *I'll exercise tomorrow.*

We have all had days like this. We mean well. We have good intentions, but when it comes right down to it, we often take care of everything else first and take care of ourselves last by neglecting our exercise. The cycle continues day in and day out until we finally ask "What changes do I need to make so I can get in my exercise?"

After 30 days of waking up early, you will have established a good habit and routine, and your natural rhythm will have you waking up sometimes before the alarm goes off.

If you feel fatigue later in the day, reward yourself with a short nap. This nap is a logical and healthy answer to taking care of ourselves, getting the exercise we need, and also getting the rest we want.

Write exercise into your daily planner or schedule of events. Even if you are a stay-at-home mom, it is important to make your exercise a priority by writing it down in your daily goals of things to do. If you do not make taking care of yourself with exercise a priority, no one else will either. Remember, exercising is more than just about taking good care of yourself. You are teaching your children and grandchildren the healthy way for them to take good care of themselves too. Actions really do speak louder than words.

Back to the Basics of Exercising

If you have never exercised, or haven't exercised in a long time, or have a medical problem, start out slowly, with five to ten minutes of exercise. You can build up to your goal a little each day by adding one minute longer to the duration of your exercise. It may sound crazy, only adding one minute more of exercise a day, but by the end of the month you'll have worked your way up to exercising for half an hour. It adds up quickly. So be gentle with yourself and give yourself time to progress without injury. It took a while to get where you are now; it'll take a little while to get into better shape. I can promise you this: You will be pleasantly surprised at how quickly your physical fitness progress will increase.

Make sure you consult with your physician before beginning any exercise program and confirm with him or her what you would like to begin doing. Physicians like being a part of a winning team, and chances are as you get closer to reaching your goals your physician will proudly share your success as your personal cheerleader. He or she will probably use your story as inspiration to encourage his or her other patients as well. Isn't it nice to know your positive influence can encourage others to strive for a better quality of life for themselves?

Preparing for an Exercise Plan

Use the right items for what you are attempting to begin— whether it's walking shoes for walking or a bike for cycling—

and make sure they are in good condition and fit you properly. Start exercising gently. Go slowly and don't try to do too much too fast or too soon. Example: Don't start lifting weights with your husband's 15-pound dumbbells unless you don't want to be able to move for a few days because you'll be too sore. Either get light weights or use my "kitchen staple" method of building your strength before investing in weights (later in this chapter).

Over and over again in my aerobic classes I've seen beginner students coming in all enthusiastic, ready to conquer the world of their unfit bodies but unrealistically thinking they were going to miraculously be transformed into a superhero physique within days. Often they would not show up to class for a week or two afterward because they were too sore. Less is more when you are starting out.

When it comes to beginning your exercise program, think like a marathon runner. You are in for the long haul, so you don't want to burst out of your exercise starting gate using all of your adrenaline like a sprint runner and have nothing left with which to finish the many miles ahead of you.

If you begin well, someday, not too long down the road, you will be amazed, maybe even shocked, at how far you have come.

K.I.S.S. Exercise Plan

You may think there is not any form of exercise you can enjoy. Oh, really? You might surprise yourself. I bet there are things you never even thought of. Look at all the wonderful forms of exercise I have listed below. Highlight the ones you enjoy. Underline exercises you have never tried but are open to trying. Wouldn't a new form of exercise you enjoy and actually look forward to be a great gift to yourself?

The number of calories burned during exercise depends on body weight, intensity of workout, conditioning level, and metabolism. Here are just a few types of exercises you might want to try and the approximate calories burned per hour for someone weighing 125, 150, 175, and 200 pounds, respectively:

Weight

	125	150	175	200
Bicycling 12 to 13.9 mph	480	576	672	768 calories
Using a stationary bike, moderate	420	504	588	672 calories
Running 12-minute miles	480	576	672	768 calories
Jumping rope	600	720	840	960 calories
Walking with 10 minutes of jogging	360	432	504	576 calories
Walking 15-minute miles	270	324	378	432 calories
Golfing, using cart	210	252	294	336 calories
Aerobics, low impact	330	396	462	528 calories
Water aerobics	240	288	336	384 calories
Swimming	360	432	504	576 calories
Weight lifting	180	216	252	288 calories

The Upside of Lifting Weights

It is very beneficial to mix cardiovascular exercise and strength training for a well-balanced, personalized program. If you have not exercised for a while, you might want to begin with just cardiovascular workouts, and then after a few weeks you can begin to add in weight training either as an add on those same days or as your alternate day's exercise.

Before you decide to invest a lot of money in weights or dumbbells, I suggest doing what I did when I first began to see if weight training was something I was interested in. Start out using lightweight cans of food, such as two cans of soup at 15 ounces each. One can be held in each hand. They can easily be returned back to the cupboard when you are finished exercising.

Do as many repetitions in a set you can comfortably do until your muscles either feel fatigued or start burning, and then do two or three more reps.

Once you are able to do up to 30 reps in a set without difficulty, increase to a heavier can or a liter of beverage, and then increase to a 2-liter beverage bottle, all the way up to a gallon jug of water. A gallon weighs eight pounds. Gallon jugs are also great for lunge exercises (if you do not have bad or weak knees).

Weight Training Tips

A "rep" is one exercise movement from beginning to end.

A "set" is numerous reps done at one time before taking a break to rest the working group of muscles. The number of reps in a set varies.

A slight burning feeling in the working muscle is okay; it's your body's way of saying it is being worked. If your muscles become so fatigued they are unable to do a rep without pain, stop immediately and shake or gently stretch the muscle until the pain subsides.

Your Personal Plan

Let's look at the type of exercises that inspire you most. Respond to these questions and then write out a sample exercise plan for one week. I encourage you to stick with this plan or make only slight modifications to it for the first month so that it becomes a healthy habit.

What are some exercises you enjoy doing?

What are exercises you have not done but are interested in giving a try?

Who are some friends you could ask to exercise with on a regular basis?

Part of the reason many people fail to exercise is because they fail to plan to exercise. Once it becomes a part of your day, your week, and your lifestyle, you will not want to miss your exercise routine.

Establishing an accountability partner increases your likelihood to sticking with your program. It is not uncommon to hear of friends who have been walking or exercising together in a certain class for years. Even though we might let ourselves down, we usually don't want to disappoint a friend, so we tend to make an extra effort to follow through with our word and be there to exercise regardless of how we feel. For those having difficulty being true to themselves, having an accountability partner can be the difference between making or breaking the goal.

Write your ideal exercise plan here. Remember, this is just your model. Most likely this original plan will be critiqued a time or two before you can iron out the wrinkles, but having an outline of the goals you'd like to achieve are imperative in knowing what direction you are headed. Set a goal to exercise for at least 30 minutes a day, five to six days a week.

Day of week	Who you'd like to exercise with	Type of exercise you'd like to do
Monday		
Tuesday		
Wednesday		
Thursday		
Friday		
Saturday		
Sunday		

Stretching Your Exercise Plan

Simple calisthenics kept bodies in shape for years before high-tech exercise and weight machines were the craze. These simple-to-follow exercises may surprise you at how challenging they can be. Use them as part of your regular exercise plan or as your form of exercise when you travel. And don't be surprised if you are a little sore for the next day or two afterward.

First start out with about five to ten minutes of stretching. Starting from your head and working your way down, hold each of these stretches for eight to ten slow counts, saying "thousand one, thousand two, thousand three," until you get to eight or ten. Each exercise you do on one side you need to do on the other side as well.

1. Standing, turn your chin as far to one shoulder as you can while pressing your shoulder down. Do your other side.

2. Hold your chin down to your chest.

3. Lift your chin as high up as you possibly can. Take your lower jaw and open and close it as wide as you can, pausing for a few counts between each movement.

4. Roll both of your shoulders at the same time, in the same direction, for ten counts.

5. Press down one shoulder as far as you can while tilting your head in the opposite direction. Repeat in other direction.

6. Bend as far forward as you possibly can, holding your hands around the back of your shins, with your legs just slightly bent so they are not locked at the knee, and allowing your head to relax as it hangs down forward.

7. Stand straight up and reach one hand, palm faced up as high over your head as you can and reach without bouncing. Do the same for the opposite side.

8. Spread your feet hip distance apart. Squat down with your hands in front of you in a frog sitting position. Gently raise your heels one at a time, holding each heel up for ten counts. Then hold both heels up at the same time for ten counts.

9. Bring your feet together and slowly sit down, wrapping your arms under your knees and around your thighs. Gently roll back and forth as far as you feel comfortable for ten counts.

10. Place your legs in front of you, and place your hands behind you with your fingers pointing away from your body. Lift your chin toward the ceiling and gently lift your pelvis up and point your toes, keeping your legs straight and feet together. Hold for ten counts.

11. Return your buttocks to the floor and spread your legs apart as far as you can comfortably stretch them. Reach the opposite hand to the opposite foot. Hold for ten counts. Repeat on the opposite side.

12. Roll over and place both elbows on the floor. Keeping your head straight, make your torso as straight as possible. Hold your lower body parallel with the floor by resting on your toes as in a military push-up stance, with your knees straight. Hold for ten counts or until you can no longer comfortably hold that stance. Lower your body to the floor. Repeat numerous times until you feel your midsection becoming weak. Then stop.

13. Roll over with your back flat on the ground. Lay your

arms next to your torso and lift your pelvis up to knee level. Squeeze your knees together as firmly as you can while holding your hips up to knee level and then release. Continue squeezing and releasing until your buttocks, hamstrings (muscles in back of upper legs), and quadriceps (muscles on top front part of legs) feel weak. Relax and lower your body.

14. Reach one leg over your body to the opposite side and have both of your arms cross in the opposite direction along with your face in the opposite direction. Hold for ten counts and repeat the opposite side.

15. Still lying down, reach both arms above your head as far as they will go. Point and flex your toes and feet as far as you can. Hold each stretch for ten counts.

The Benefits of Exercise

Exercise...

■ reduces anxiety and depression and is a natural mood lifter

■ helps you handle stress better

■ helps control your weight

■ helps control joint swelling and pain from arthritis

■ gives you more energy throughout the day

■ helps you sleep better

■ helps you feel better about yourself

- lowers your risk of dying from heart disease, cancer, diabetes, and stroke

- lowers your risk of getting heart disease, stroke, high blood pressure, colon cancer, and diabetes

- lowers high blood pressure

- helps keep your bones, muscles, and joints healthy and less achy

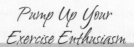

*Pump Up Your
Exercise Enthusiasm*

Exercise with different friends on different days of the week.

Create a backup plan for yucky weather days when you can't exercise outside.

Have a variety of exercise videos or DVDs you enjoy.

Do different forms of exercising on different days.

Share videos or DVDs of different types of exercise with your friends and family members or borrow them from the library.

Try a 12-week class by an instructor you've never had or in an exercise of interest that you've always wanted to try.

Read a good book or pop in a good movie to help time pass while on the treadmill, stair stepper, or stationary bike.

Listen to various types of music with headphones during exercise.

The Satisfied Life

People who are passionate about running describe the feeling they get mid-activity as a "runner's high." As the body works like the efficient machine of flesh, bone, and muscle that it is, there is a feeling of great satisfaction. We might not all pursue marathons or run sprints around the neighborhood, but any of us can relate to this sense of accomplishment when we stick to an exercise plan.

Give yourself the gift of this sensation. It might not happen the first week, or even the second—when your body is sore and you don't want to get up early to walk or do the exercise DVD that started out as being fun. But somewhere after this time of creating a routine, you will discover satisfaction in the discipline of living fully and treating yourself and your body with respect. This is a natural high that does not require special shoes or a race registration fee. And these glimpses of satisfaction and self-worth will inspire you on the days when your passion needs a boost.

Devotional Health

Exercise your inner strength muscles by spending time alone with God. Maybe add a devotional time to your scheduled exercise so that you can be encouraged by faith and energized by God's faithfulness. Consider doing your Bible reading while on the treadmill. Large-print Bibles and devotional books work great. Many exercises, such as walking or using the cardio machines at the gym, give us plenty of time to think lots of thoughts and work through our feelings. Spend a few moments after you are finished working out to pray about what surfaced in your mind and heart during this time of physical effort. You will find this spiritual exercise to be an exhilarating part of your new routine.

Prayer

God, help me make a commitment to myself and to this body You created. Encourage me to see how it was made to move and grow strong. Your hand formed me in my mother's womb. When I ignore my health, I am rejecting the miracle of me. When I don't think I am worth the effort, I am denying the potential You planted inside of me. And when I spend time wallowing in frustration over my body or my life, I am holding myself back from ways to be whole and serve You. Help me choose to make exercise a priority in my life. Amen.

*Complete the Step Four page
of your Personal Plan for a Healthier Me
at the back of the book.*

Step 5 | De-Clutter Your Life

Often it is easier to blame somebody or something else for the state we are in, rather than being painfully honest about the role we've played in our well-being. When we blame others for our state of being, we relinquish power and control over our own lives and play the role of victim vs. that of overcomer. Until a few years ago, I was great at caring for others, but myself...that was another story. I think part of it was an unhealthy interpretation on my part as to what God expected from me. All I could focus on was serving others, but God wants balance, which includes taking time for me as well.

The Bible says, "Do you not know that your body is

a temple of the Holy Spirit, who is in you, whom you have received from God? You are not your own; you were bought at a price. Therefore honor God with your body" (1 Corinthians 6:19-20).

The temple of God can also be considered the house of God. This being the case, don't you agree that some of our houses need cleaning out and de-cluttering? When I say houses, I am referring not only to our physical body, but our entire being: our heart, mind, thoughts, and spirit as well.

Purifying and de-cluttering ourselves inside and out is an important part of becoming healthy, happy, and whole. We can easily say that we want this, but if we stick to unhealthy habits, no change will take place. The transformation will remain an unattainable goal. I write the *Busy People's* cookbooks. What if I want to create a new recipe but use the exact same ingredients and cooking instructions from another recipe? What if I did this over and over, hoping for a different result? Fat chance, right? Only a fool would use the same ingredients and hope for different results. For different results, we need to do things differently.

It can be difficult for people to let go of things they don't want to let go of, even bad things. On the one hand, they want to clear away obstacles to their goals, but on the other hand, they depend on clutter to distract them from what is important. A way to clear out junk, distractions, and misleading priorities is to focus solely on what needs to be done. It goes back to being very intentional in your efforts. This step will help you figure out what needs to go and what needs to stay in your life in order for you to be healthy.

It is difficult to completely de-clutter your home and life of things that are robbing you of the opportunity to be your best you. Let's face it. Often we like sugar instead of healthy food choices. We like staying up late and watching TV instead of going to sleep at a decent time. We like sleeping in rather than getting up to exercise.

Write down things you know you want to get rid of to de-clutter your home and life so you have room for healthier choices.

What things are you holding on to that are not serving you well?

What things are you holding on to that are holding you back from being who you want to be?

Take a walk through your house and observe time or energy traps. Maybe go around several times because at first you won't notice every obstacle. It is the casual pile of books on the floor by the couch that you have stepped over for months. It is the bedroom door that squeaks all day long as the wind blows through the hallway. It is the bag of items you meant to give away to a local charity last season. It is the file drawer that overflows with folders marked "to file later." It is the doctor's appointment you were supposed to make several months ago.

These bits and pieces of clutter can really affect your well-being. Not one of them is a disaster, or even a huge hindrance, but these annoyances can pile up. Or the things that never get done become a weight on your shoulders that you are not able to shake. Take an inventory of such pieces in your home and in your life. Give yourself a plan that will become a part of your weekly schedule. Maybe you want to start with one hour a week or 20 minutes a day to tend to these small projects.

The amazing part about this effort is that it will inspire you. It will clear your head and mind and reenergize your life as tasks are taken care of—as the work of life is done with intentional effort and the desire for a life that makes room for beauty, fulfillment, peace, and the space for new goals and new ways of looking at your home, your family, your body, your faith, and your future.

Losing the Weight of Temptation

You are moving toward more exercise. You are changing your meal plan to provide your body with valuable fuel. You are connecting with others so that you have support. Now comes one of the most helpful and difficult steps. We are going to de-fat and de-sugar your home. Take a garbage bag and literally throw away all of the junk food, high-processed, high-sugar foods that are hard for you to resist. You don't need them and they are holding you back.

You may have made the commitment to avoid these temptations, but I'll bet you will face some resistance from your family once they see that it is sugar cereal and not broccoli that is going into that garbage sack. But your kids don't need these foods either. Maybe there are a few treats you want to keep around for the occasional movie night or special dessert for your family—it is fine to keep these on hand, but only if they do not get in the way of your success. Only you can make the decision.

If you have children, include them in the process of selecting healthy snacks to fill the void of the absent sugar. Choose an afternoon to have a taste test of unique fruits, vegetables, yogurts, and healthy crackers. Select the winners and declare them a household approved snack. Every month or every other month have another taste test and include those fruits and vegetables that are in season. A great way to get friends or family excited about healthy choices is to plan a weekend day to go to local produce and berry farms for a good old-fashioned day of harvesting. The fruit of your labor will be that much sweeter.

As you clear out the temptations from your house, consider your danger zone people and places and your backup plans. How are you arranging your days or activities to accommodate those backup plans?

These small changes will begin to change your life in bigger ways. You will discover that taking care of yourself has many wonderful benefits for you and the people you love most. After a few weeks of this effort, take a moment to ask "If someone observed my life before and my life now, would they notice a difference?" If the answer is no, you are still deciding if you are worth the effort. If the answer is yes, then congratulations. You have a foundation for a healthy new you.

Stinkin' Thinking—The Junk Food of the Mind

"Out with the bad, in with the good." This can be your mantra for all aspects of your life. You will notice, as the process of change begins in your life, that you think through choices very deliberately. After you have fed yourself comfort food for years, it is not easy to switch your junk food tendencies or stinkin' thinking junk food thoughts.

These negative thoughts do not nourish you or provide you with energy to move you forward. They provide a bit of comfort in some way, but only because you are used to the presence of these complaints or negative ideas. Have you ever stopped to identify your stinkin' thinking junk food thoughts? If you want to bring a few to the surface, imagine trying on bathing suits at the mall. All kinds of stinkin' thinking thoughts emerge. Or how about even some of the self-defeating thoughts you have had while working through these steps?

Write down some of your whoppers…your most common stinkin' thinking junk food thoughts.

When do these thoughts pop into your mind? Write out where you usually are or what the typical circumstance is that triggers these thoughts.

Stinkin' thinking thoughts affect how we think of ourselves, others, and our efforts toward change. Before they can taint your desire for a new way of living, go through the following exercise. These are deliberately different ways to think of food choices. After reading through my versions, try a few of your own. Don't just limit this elimination of junk food thinking to your food decisions, but also include how these fatty thoughts enter your mind when you face exercise, positive change, or even a challenge that will inspire personal growth.

Trade in:

Potato chips for cucumber slices lightly salted with low-sodium salt or flavored popcorn salt. *"I'd much rather have these crunchy cucumbers than those fatty potato chips I used to eat. I feel so much healthier when I replace healthier crunchy food for unhealthy crunchy chips.*

High-fat sour cream for fat-free sour cream. *I love knowing I can eat the same amount. I am saving 40 calories simply by substituting fat-free sour cream instead of high-fat regular sour cream and am not missing the fat in the flavor. Life is good.*

Regular crackers for fat-free or low-fat crackers. *I can't believe I didn't switch to eating fat-free crackers long ago. They taste so good. I actually think they taste better.*

High-fat hamburger for ground eye of round. *This ground eye of round beef is so much leaner. It's not greasy like my old hamburgers. I can actually taste the beef.*

High-fat hamburger for ground meatless vegetarian crumbles. *Okay, I was surprised, but this is really good in spaghetti sauce, chili, and taco meat. I love how easy it is to cook with because I don't have to pre-brown it first, and I know my family will never taste the difference.*

High-fat or low-fat Italian turkey sausage cooked and crumbled for vegetarian sausage crumbles. *I cannot believe how delicious these vegetarian sausage crumbles are in omelets, casseroles, and soups. It saves me so much time, fat, and calories. It's unbelievable, and the flavor is fabulous.*

Regular salad dressing for fat-free salad dressings. *Salad dressings have come a long way. These taste so good, I don't know why I ever ate the high-fat dressings and wasted all those calories for nothing.*

Breakfast sausage for low-fat breakfast sausage links. *These are really good, especially in casseroles and breakfast scrambles or sausage gravy over biscuits. Who'd ever know you could eat so well and have low fat too?*

High-fat cheeses for fat-free cheeses. *These fat-free cheeses taste good when they are mixed in with other ingredients because they absorb the flavor from the other ingredients and aren't rubbery. I also like low-fat cheese on a burger. All I have to do is turn my hamburger over in the skillet and put the cheese on, cover with a lid and let the moisture from the meat melt the cheese to make it creamy.*

Regular Popsicles for fat-free, sugar-free Popsicles. *These taste even better than the regular Popsicles, and I can have four of these sugar-free ones for the same amount of calories in a single regular treat.*

High-fat butter for half-fat butter: *This is too good to believe. I am eating real, creamy butter and I absolutely love the taste, and it is only half the calories of the regular high-fat butter. Thank You, God.*

Oil in cooking and baking for nonfat cooking sprays. *Why have I been adding all that unnecessary fat to our family's food for no reason at all? This spray is so super easy.*

White bread for low-carb bread or low-calorie bread. *It is amazing that I can have two slices of this low-carb bread for the same amount of calories in one slice of regular white bread, and this healthier bread is so much more filling and satisfying. I like that I am getting extra fiber too.*

Bologna, salami, and other high-fat lunch meats for lean ham, turkey, or roast beef. *I can't believe how much more meat I get for so much less fat and calories by switching from bologna.*

Regular high-fat mayonnaise and regular Miracle Whip for reduced fat or fat-free mayonnaise and light or fat-free Miracle Whip. *I cannot tell the difference at all in the reduced-fat Miracle Whip or reduced-fat salad dressing on my sandwiches. I'd rather eat the lower fat than the fat free because I can tell a big difference in the fat-free compared to the lower fat when it is on my sandwiches, and the difference is only three grams of fat. However, in salads, when the fat-free Miracle Whip and the fat-free salad dressings are mixed with other ingredients, I can't tell them apart from the high fat, so I've made the switch and I'll never go back.*

Stillness in the Busyness

Our lives are filled with busyness, noise, distractions, and many thoughts that fill our minds and crowd out our peace. The practice of stillness will encourage you to de-clutter your mind and prepare yourself for purposeful living.

When is the last time you stopped to breathe? I mean breathe in and breathe out in a conscious manner? When you can practice the kind of breathing that allows you to count the breaths and track the air as it fills your lungs and gives your body energy and flows back out, taking with it stress and internal clutter, then you will be closer to stillness.

Most women I talk to envision the practice of stillness to be something that involves hours of meditation or yoga mats and candles, with instrumental music in the background. Well, that could be one of your healthy choices, but this detailed scene and the significant amount of time is not required for you to reap the benefits of what I call "easy breathing."

Do you spend a lot of time in the car? I find myself taking my kids here and there and running errands much more often than I would care to admit. And while all this driving can take a big toll on your energy, you will discover that it also affords you some moments to practice stillness.

I used to become impatient while waiting for my girls to get out of school. Whether the weather was hot or cold, I would feel a slow burn rising up inside of me because I felt I was wasting time I could not spare. But what I was really doing was wasting energy and emotions along with time because of the way I used that time.

There are healthy ways to wait for someone or something. Now I practice easy breathing and take a few moments to feel the gift of the quiet time. I take in a large amount of air to fill my lungs, stretch them, and let them feel the renewal of oxygen. Instead of being frustrated or anxious, I become prayerful. My thoughts go to people who need prayer, or I end up praising God for my family, my health, and even the time of waiting.

Whether your clutter is tangible or emotional, it can rise up and create a wall around you. It can choke you. It can steal away the gift of change. Stillness and the discipline of evaluating hurtful habits will tear down those walls, restore you, and inspire change. It is as easy as breathing.

The Satisfied Life

We feel great satisfaction after cleaning a room,

organizing a kitchen, or giving away a pile of clothes to someone who can use them. We don't always want to do the work to get the dust-free room, the orderly kitchen, or the roomy closet, but when we push through the excuses and the distractions and roll up our sleeves, it is mighty satisfying. Think about how you can clean your mental house. Maybe there is a room where you tuck every put-down or insult you ever received or imagined you received. There is probably a closet-sized space where you stack past mistakes. You might even have an office where you carefully label your wrongdoings. Pick any of these places and start purging this unnecessary, energy-stealing stuff. Replace anything you remove with promises of health and vitality. And replenish your mental home with the promises of God.

_____ Devotional Health _____

Face off with your junk food cupboard or drawer. We all have them. If you are not ready for the garbage bag activity, at least clear out those items which are your biggest downfall. Ask for others to provide you with strength. Take time this week to consider which tasks or activities seem to steal your energy. How can that change? Journal a note to God asking Him to open your eyes to those things, people, and places that cause you to stumble.

Prayer _____

Lord, I keep tripping over the same things in my life. The same bad habits or unhealthy choices rise up and block my progress. Give me eyes to see how I repeat the old patterns which undermine my new efforts. Give me a glimpse of the freedom that comes with being healthy and whole. Amen.

> *Complete the Step Five page of your Personal Plan for a Healthier Me at the back of the book.*

Step 6 | Get Spiritually Fit

God has a plan and a purpose for your life, and it includes more love, joy, peace, serenity, and good health than you could have ever imagined.

The number one key to having and enjoying God's ultimate best for you in all aspects of your life, including body, mind, and spirit, is to make God number one in your life.

Faith and Faithfulness

Having faith allows us to practice faithfulness in our lives. When we know what unconditional love and complete trust look like, we can create these things in our own relationships, whether that is with our spouse, our friends, or even our own bodies. Becoming spiritually fit strengthens the muscles of our commitment, discipline, and resolve because we learn the promise of faithfulness. As we grow closer to God, we witness the goodness that comes with trusting our Creator.

These are all vital steps that stretch your heart and spirit and allow you to achieve the spiritual fitness you need for overall good health:

- Make the decision to live healthier and recommit to it daily.

- Be honest with yourself.

- Stay totally focused on God and His will for you.

- Allow God to do for you and through you what you have been unable to do on your own.

- Be obedient and follow through with your part by doing what you say you are going to do: have a daily plan and follow through with it regardless of how you feel.

- Check in with God on a regular basis throughout the day. Ask Him what it is He wants from you and make Him accountable for your success.

- Take one day at a time. When times are tough, take one moment at a time.

- Replace negative thoughts with positive thoughts of thanks for the many blessings you have.

- Believe you can make changes through God's strength.

Take time to be quiet and reflect about your life. If you

answer any of the following questions with "I don't know," then give the question to God. He knows and will give you the wisdom you seek.

This inward search for truth and knowledge is every bit as important (if not more so) than physical exercising. Consider making this effort to recharge your spiritual batteries. Unless you take time for this as a top priority, you will not make progress.

Is God number one in your life?

If not, what is number one in your life?

What holds you back from having God's complete fullness of love, joy, peace, prosperity, and good health?

What are some choices you need to make in order to begin your first steps toward wholeness in body?

What are some choices you need to make in order to begin your first steps toward wholeness in mind?

What are some choices you need to make in order to begin your first steps toward wholeness in spirit?

True Will Power

Some people are happy being unhappy and content being discontent. Often these people grew up in unhealthy circumstances and are more comfortable feeling uncomfortable. Others desire to feel good but do not have the personal strength to motivate themselves, to inspire change, or to believe in what is possible for them.

Unless we admit there is an area of our life that is not completely healthy, we cannot recover in that area. Improving ourselves is a lifelong journey that begins only when we want it to. It is a growing and learning process that will continue the rest of our lives.

Often people nonchalantly say they don't have the will power. I wonder if a lack of will power or a lack of a plan is really responsible for defeat when it comes to good health or any other goal.

There is a difference between wanting something enough to work for it and wanting something in a "it would be nice, but not worth my effort" way. The questions to ask are:

How important is this to you?

Why do you want it?

How much do you want it?

What price are you willing to pay of your time, energy, and effort for it?

God gives us freedom of choice. He will give us the help we need if we ask Him to help us, yet He allows us the freedom to ask for help. As my father-in-law says, "God helps those who help themselves." Living a healthier lifestyle is a perfect example of this saying in action.

When actual will power is a problem, thank goodness we are not asked to rely solely on our will power to create change and experience transformation.

Pray for God's will for your life, knowledge of it, and strength to carry it through. Sometimes we feel frustrated with the amount of will power we have because we try to accomplish things we want solely with our own strength. We can seek God's best for our lives. We know He wants good health for us, among a multitude of other blessings, but does God really want you to be a certain number on the scale or a certain pant size that is always frustrating for you to obtain and maintain or is that what you want? Does God care if you are unhealthy? Yes, because He wants you to be healthy. Does God care if you wear a size 8 or a size 6? I think not.

God is more concerned with the size of our spiritual and emotional hearts than He is the size of our clothes.

What is *God's will* for my lifestyle in regard to eating and exercise?

Am I living the healthy lifestyle I know God wants me to live?

Am I putting too much thought, energy, and frustration into what the scale says daily?

If so, why?

Is there some lesson God wants me to learn? If so, what is it?

What do I need to change with my eating habits in order to be in line with God's will for me physically?

If you are living a healthy lifestyle and have a negative body image, I want to encourage you. Your negative body image will heal as you get closer in your relationship with God, and you will become more grateful for the good health you have, you will become more confident, and you will have more self-esteem.

Once we really know what God's will is for our healthy lifestyle, it is important that we obey, write down exactly what we are to do, and do not set ourself up for failure.

We all know that our will power does not emerge when we are hungry, tired, and wandering around the grocery store looking for something to eat at the last moment. Nor does will power to do exercise kick in when we are tired at the end of the day and contemplating *What should I do for exercise today?* We can increase our will power by planning ahead and by eliminating as many temptations as possible.

To say "I have no will power" is to say "I have no inner strength." To have no inner strength is the total opposite of what God says He gives us. Over and over the Bible tells us how God strengthens us when we seek His help. Isn't it comforting to know that, though we were once weak and felt we had no will power, there is hope and we don't have to go through this challenge of living a healthier lifestyle alone? God will be our strength and our help in time of need. "The LORD is my strength and my shield; my heart trusts in him, and I am helped" (Psalm 28:7). Trusting in His presence and His love will carry us and protect us.

So how much is the quality of your life worth to you? You know God's will for you is to have the best. What about you? Are you willing to accept God's will for you to have and enjoy the best, or are you willing to settle for less?

Sometimes accepting God's will for your life and making the changes you know He wants you to make can feel very awkward at first. Here's a good example. Try this: Hold your hands together, intertwining your fingers. Take notice of which thumb is on top. Now hold your hands together again, this time putting the opposite thumb on top. Notice how awkward it feels. As you make significant changes in your life, it may feel awkward for you to experience God's will of fullness of love, joy, peace, prosperity, and good health if you are not accustomed to it.

Will it be challenging at times? Most likely, yes. Will it feel awkward at times? Probably. The transition of doing what you know God wants you to do compared to your old way of life—doing what *you feel* like, when *you feel* like it—may be so challenging and difficult that you might feel you aren't the same person. That means you are growing and becoming more of the person God wants you to be, and the rewards will be far greater than you have ever thought of, dreamed of, or imagined.

You will be amazed at your transformation. You will be in awe of the rewards you will receive and enjoy because of your obedience to doing what God wants you to do. When you are living in God's will for your life, you will be in awe of the energy you have to do things that at one time just the thought of overwhelmed you and seemed impossible. You will be shocked at the results. You'll wonder why you never turned your will over to God's care sooner.

Without God being number one in our life and without living in His will, we can never be or have all that He has for us. It is physically impossible. It is only when we tap into the supernatural spiritual energies of God (our Creator and Redeemer), that we can live a supernatural existence here on earth. I call it living in the flow of God.

Maybe you have tried more times than you care to count to lose that excess fat and get in better shape. Maybe you feel it is useless; you are sick and tired of trying. I encourage you: Don't give up hope. God can do through you what you have been unable to do on your own, if and when you are ready and willing to hand your life and your will over to His care.

I see miracles happen all the time. Don't put God in a box. I see lives changed for the better every day. Why not allow yourself the privilege of tapping into God's endless resources and start living the healthier, happier life you know He has in store for you?

Trusting His Word

The transformation you hope for will begin in your heart and spirit. Trusting in God's promises will lead you when you are lost, comfort you when you long for food, fill you when you are hungry for affirmation, and complete you when you feel less than perfect.

Feed on the Word of God and let it nourish you today.

> He humbled you, causing you to hunger and then feeding you with manna, which neither you nor your fathers had known, to teach you that man does not live on bread alone but on every word that comes from the mouth of the LORD (Deuteronomy 8:3).

> The LORD is righteous in all his ways and loving toward all he has made. The LORD is near to all who call on him, to all who call on him in truth (Psalm 145:17-18).

> I will refresh the weary and satisfy the faint (Jeremiah 31:25).

> You still the hunger of those you cherish; their

sons have plenty, and they store up wealth for their children (Psalm 17:14).

Because your love is better than life, my lips will glorify you (Psalm 63:3).

The laborer's appetite works for him; his hunger drives him on (Proverbs 16:26).

Teach me to do your will, for you are my God; may your good Spirit lead me on level ground (Psalm 143:10).

Look to the LORD and his strength; seek his face always (1 Chronicles 16:11).

You have made known to me the path of life; you will fill me with joy in your presence, with eternal pleasures at your right hand (Psalm 16:11).

Satisfy us in the morning with your unfailing love, that we may sing for joy and be glad all our days (Psalm 90:14).

Blessed are those who hunger and thirst for righteousness, for they will be filled (Matthew 5:6)

O LORD, hear my prayer, listen to my cry for mercy; in your faithfulness and righteousness come to my relief (Psalm 143:1).

Test me, O LORD, and try me, examine my heart and my mind; for your love is ever before me, and I walk continually in your truth (Psalm 26:2-3).

The Satisfied Life

Spiritual fitness is the key to contentment. It is never about settling for less than God calls you to. It is also never about exchanging His views for the world's perspective of joy and peace. You see, the world will sell you a big line about happiness, but it is based on tangibles, disposables, and reproachable things. But God does not sell us anything. He brings us along and makes us spiritually stronger and wiser if we are open to it. And this journey leads to a contentment that does not depend on the market or the trends. Pure contentment is born out of a peace that takes deep root within and cannot be disturbed by life's ups and downs. It is an ever-present, lasting force in a satisfied life.

Devotional Health

Take time to read and reread the verses in this chapter. Meditate on them and select one or a couple to be your key verses during your journey toward health. Or if there is a verse that inspires you that is not on this list, add it to the others.

Prayer

Lord, may I seek Your face when I hunger for validation, for love, for a reason to live life fully. Use my days and shape them to suit Your will and not my own. When I am tempted to wander from the path You have set before me, reveal to me the way I need to go. I trust in You, and it is Your will that holds me up and leads me on. Amen.

*Complete the Step Six page
of your Personal Plan for a Healthier Me
at the back of the book.*

Step 7 | Commit to the New Lifestyle

Great are the demands of being a woman. We might be a daughter, sister, granddaughter, wife, mother, stepmother, aunt, volunteer, employee, children's chauffeur, caregiver, manager, accounts payable clerk, cook, cleaning lady, gift buyer, grocery shopper, repair person, nurse, counselor, and many other roles we adopt and make our own. This is why step seven is so important. Committing to yourself and a new lifestyle while also juggling these other roles will be the truest test of your transformation.

While playing out these roles and making our way through our life, danger zones will pop up when our defenses are down.

And these places of possible distraction from our commitment to new priorities are everyday places or settings, including our cars, movies, restaurants, social gatherings, grocery shopping, and other perfectly normal circumstances.

K.I.S.S. Survival Plans

In the Car

Because we can spend a large part of our day in the car driving to and from work or events or our children's activities, this is one of the places where our boredom or stress will manifest in unhealthy choices. To counter this possible response to idle time in a vehicle, I suggest you keep some snacks in the car on a regular basis. And if it is a day when the children and you will be in the car for long stretches of time, I recommend that you bring a small cooler so that beverages and other healthy snacks will be kept fresh and within reach.

You might think that this makes the snacks too available. But these wise options will keep us from hitting drive-through restaurants, the market, or the snack shack at sports events. Let's face it. When we have had a long day running errands, working, and looking after our families, and the children are in the backseat suggesting fast food, it is easy to give in because it can sound mighty good to us as well when our defenses are down.

These K.I.S.S. survival tips will help us stay committed to the healthier life. The following are items I have in the trunk of my car:

bottled water	rice cakes
beef jerky	fruit
protein bars	sugarless gum and
low-fat granola bars	candy

At Entertainment or Sporting Events

For those of us who have a hard time resisting freshly popped, lightly salted, buttery popcorn that makes our mouth water, the movie theater can be one of the most important places to come prepared with healthier snack choices. Fruit or fruit roll ups might be a possibility. If you set aside a special day to have movie popcorn, get a smaller size and request this without the butter. It is still an indulgence, but at least you are setting limits on how much you will consume and how many calories it will have.

If you ever take your children to the circus, amusement parks, the zoo, or sporting events, you know what awaits you—many overpriced unhealthy temptations. This is when that stash in the car comes in handy.

Also, make your homemade version of snack time fun for you and the family by eating picnic style or selecting favorite treats like dips for vegetable sticks or frozen yogurt pops or a healthy trail mix with nuts, raisins, dried cranberries, and maybe a little chocolate.

What other events or activities entice you with junk food or sugar-filled treats? Write a list. On the left write the location of temptation, in the middle column list the unhealthy temptations. Next to it write a realistic, simple substitution you discretely can bring with you instead.

Example:

Location	Unhealthy Temptation	Back-up Plan/ Substitution
Movie theaters	Movie theatre popcorn	low-fat popcorn (single serving size)

At Restaurants

Eating in our own homes where we have removed many if not all of the temptations is much easier on us than dining at restaurants. The good news is that when you make a few simple decisions before you go out to eat, the restaurant experience can give you a break from cooking and a chance to eat as healthy as ever.

If you are involved in selecting the restaurant, choose one that offers vegetable dishes or lean meats and healthy side dishes. When you go to casual places, you might be able to order breakfast all day, which can be healthy with eggs, and dry whole wheat toast, and juices or filling meals like oatmeal. Just watch out for too many extras like cheese or sauces.

Practicing portion control can actually be easy at restaurants if you stand up for yourself initially by asking questions about the size of certain dishes or what extras might come with the meal that would tempt you. Some women don't even look at the menu; instead, they ask the waiter or waitress specifically for something healthy, such as a salad with low-fat dressing on the side or a steamed vegetable dish with rice or a broth-based soup.

The pleasure of eating out is possible for someone who is choosing to eat healthy. Going to different ethnic restaurants can also introduce you to how other cultures prepare healthy foods like vegetables, soups, and salads.

Parties and Other Events

Special events such as weddings, showers, and other cele-brations like family or high school reunions can lead us down a path of weakness.

These occasions often trigger more than emotional eating—they can trigger the "buffet syndrome," which causes us to plow through a buffet table without any sense of time, portions, or control. It is as if the long rows of platters, plates, bowls, and flower-shaped radishes override any of our rational arguments for sticking to our program.

Here are some helpful ideas which I call "buffet buffers." If you still want to hurdle the other women and children in line to get to salmon pate, you will. But if you follow these suggestions, you might not reach that point of desperation.

1. While everyone else goes to the buffet, go to the restroom or quiet area to spend that time praying or relaxing. Visit with others who haven't gotten their food yet. This will not only help you prepare your mind, body, and spirit, but also be a practical way for you to have less time to eat without having the food staring you in the face while everyone else is eating.

2. Try to be helpful in getting the children's plates prepared. The more time you divert your mind on other things, the less time you have to be concerned about all of the tasty foods you want to try to avoid.

3. Go to the restroom to wash your hands in order to avoid immediately stepping in the food line. Without being obvious to others, this is another way to help use up time we would normally spend eating.

4. Before walking up to the buffet, ask yourself, *What food sounds really good to eat right now? What am I craving?* The answer to this question will help give you focus as you approach a wide assortment of options. It can also keep you from wandering around areas of the

buffet that will tempt you to eat things you shouldn't. Remember, it is easier to avoid than resist. So take the long way around the table to avoid the dessert area unless you have planned your meal around that treat.

5. Ask yourself, *Will I be allowing myself to have a taste or two of anything that is not considered healthy food, such as a fried food or dessert?* Answering this question in advance before approaching the buffet acknowledges the agreement you are making with yourself before you start choosing the foods you are about to eat.

6. While at the buffet you have two helpful methods for selecting and eating. Choose a little bit of a lot of different foods you can taste a bite or two of or allow yourself a bit larger portions of two to three different healthy proteins and carbohydrates—all combined totaling about one and a half times the size of your fist—and as many fresh or steamed vegetables as you'd like.

7. Stay focused on the foods you are enjoying and have selected, not what other people are eating. A definite sign of food addiction is when we do what I call "food patrol," watching and keeping track of what others are eating instead of focusing on ourselves. Often food patrol syndrome happens when we feel deprived or jealous.

At Grocery Stores

Most grocery stores and even the food markets inside superstores are laid out similarly, and they all have their own danger zones for any of us. The outside perimeter of the supermarket is usually the safe zone. Visualize your grocery store. When you first walk in, the produce areas are often to the side, and then the meats and fresh dairy are followed by whole grains and baked goods.

The inside aisles are the danger zone, full of processed and junk foods such as snacks, chips, cookies, candy, sugar-laden sodas, and juices.

The key is to focus on where you want to be in the store and stay away from tempting areas. We have all heard the advice to eat before shopping so your stomach does not cause you to overshop. We also benefit by planning before we shop as well. Which sections do you need to visit? What is on your grocery list? Head into the store with your plan in mind or in hand. There's no need to roam the aisles. Lots of women do this to spot the sale items, but it is difficult to see a three for $5.00 sale on your favorite cookies and pass them up. This is not a bargain because it will cost you your healthy lifestyle.

Choose Well

Healthy eating doesn't begin with what you eat; it begins with what you purchase to eat (and in the choices we make prior to our actual first bite). So choosing well is very key to your success.

If you choose well, you won't end up going home with foods that have zero fat and zero taste and eventually end up in the round cupboard—the wastebasket. My motto regarding low-fat and low-carb foods is "If it doesn't taste good, don't eat it." There are too many delicious choices available today for any of us to waste calories on food that doesn't taste good.

The following lists are products I enjoy using. Here's an easy rule of thumb when reading labels: If it has more than 3 grams of fat per 100 calories, don't buy it. When it comes to healthy foods, the only times I break that rule is for half-fat butter, which I like on toast, and also you can have more than 3 grams of fat for super lean beef and pork such as:

Type of Beef	Serving Size	Fat Grams	Calories	% Fat Calories
London Broil/Flank Steak	3 oz.	6	167	32%
Top Loin (Lean Only)	3 oz.	6	162	33%
Eye of Round (As a steak, roast, or have butcher grind for superlean hamburger)	3 oz.	5	150	30%

I encourage you to make the switch to ground eye of round if you enjoy eating red meat and do not want to refrain. You'll be doing your heart, health, and waistline a lot of good.

Staples

Here's an easy-to-follow list of lighter food choices for staples:

high-fiber breads and buns

enriched flour

fat-free flour tortillas

graham crackers

Health Valley fat-free cookies

Health Valley fat-free granola

Italian-seasoned bread crumbs

light breads with no more than 40 calories per slice

Nabisco reduced-fat crackers

oyster crackers

pastas (except egg noodles; pastas from whole durum wheat or brown rice are best)

rice cakes

rice (whole grain or brown)

vegetable bread

whole wheat flour

whole grain breads

low-fat cheeses

soups

beans

eggs (use only the whites)

egg substitute

Condiments

Here are just a few of my favorites. You will find that adding spices and vegetables will be the better way to dress a dish with extra flavor. Check labels of your favorite condiments. If one of the top few ingredients is sugar, try to find a substitute. (Note: Because all oils—even olive oil—are very calorie dense, I try to avoid adding oil, even olive oil.)

low-fat salad dressings (they spruce up salad and also can be great marinades)

taco seasoning mixes

honey

sea salt

nonsalt seasonings

tomato sauce instead of a cream sauce for pasta and other
   meals

ketchup (check ingredients)

soy sauce

mustard

sugar substitutes (such as Splenda)

plain yogurt as a substitute for sour cream

applesauce (this can be great in recipes as a natural
   sweetener)

Butter Buds

half-fat butter

butter-flavored and nonfat cooking sprays

Snacks

The first preference for a snack should be fruits and
vegetables. But now and then you and your family are going to
have a need for a crunchy, zesty, or tangy treat. Here are some
good options to have on hand:

baked chips

salsa

rice cakes

popcorn (low fat, lightly salted)

pretzels

fruit or juice bars

Popsicles (low sugar)

real fruit-flavored yogurt

wheat crackers (low fat)

rice crackers

Meats, Fish, Poultry

beef (tenderloin, eye of round, London broil, flank steak, top loin)

Butterball low-fat sausage

turkey breast and lunch meats

Canadian bacon (usually very low fat)

bouillon cubes (chicken, beef, vegetable)

chicken breast (no skin; dark meat has twice as much fat)

crab meat (imitation or real)

Eckrich fat-free meats (hot dogs, lunch meats, smoked sausage, kielbasa)

fish (the white ones are lower in fats; i.e., flounder, grouper, pike, sole, cod, orange roughy, monk fish, perch, scallops)

Healthy Choice lunch meat, hot dogs, and smoked sausage

Hillshire Farms low-fat smoked sausage and kielbasa

Morningstar ground meatless vegetarian meat substitute (for chili, pasta sauce, etc., but not alone as a burger)

shellfish (lobster, crab, shrimp)

tuna (packed in water)

Fruits and Veggies

organic when possible or fresh from a local farm

canned vegetables (no salt added)

canned fruits in fruit juice only

fresh vegetables—all (except for avocado—major fat)

frozen vegetables and fruits—all (with no sugar added)

light fruit cocktail

light pie fillings—cherry, apple, blueberry, strawberry, peach

Healthy, Not Wealthy

Sometimes low-fat, fat-free, or low-carb products are more expensive than high-fat, high-carb products. I am a frugal person, so this is not often easy to swallow. But there are ways to still save on your healthy choices.

One way I've saved about 30 percent on my groceries without using coupons is to make a list of the products I like to use often. I did a price comparison of what stores have the lowest prices on certain items. I found that certain stores consistently sold certain products at a lower price than others. Knowing this made my job a whole lot easier. Now I regularly purchase certain products at certain stores at the overall lowest price found locally. When I see a product on sale for less than I normally pay, I usually get it and stock up.

Take time to comparison shop. Make a list of the products you purchase most often. List the three to four stores you shop most often. I know for sure to purchase gift bags at the dollar store for $1.00 each on big bags or two for $1.00 on medium size bags. I buy boneless skinless chicken breast for not more than $1.99 a pound; for my favorite soft, high-quality toilet paper I never pay more than 25 cents a roll. And my favorite name-brand laundry fabric softener is never more than 10 cents a load.

In order to shop wisely and get more for your money, you need to know what the going rate is for that product.

Here's a miniature example of my chart.

Item	Store 1	Store 2	Store 3	Store 4
Frozen veggies	0.89	1.20	1.00	0.79
Canned veggies	0.50	.78	N/A	0.29
Chicken breast	1.99	3.99	2.50	2.30
Eye of round	2.49	3.99	4.29	N/A
Promise margarine	1.89	1.69	N/A	N/A
Healthy Choice cheese	2.39	1.99	N/A	N/A
Film developing (36 exp.)	6.20	5.10	3.24	N/A
Eggs—1 dozen	0.75	1.09	0.80	0.60
Skim milk	2.29	1.89	1.89	1.89
Low-sugar, fat-free yogurt	0.35	0.69	0.50	0.29
Baked Lays potato chips	3.29	3.39	2.49	N/A
Baked Tostitos	3.59	3.31	2.69	N/A
Fat-free frozen yogurt	1.89	4.99	3.99	N/A

Make your own chart (fill in store names).

Item	Store 1	Store 2	Store 3	Store 4
1.				
2.				
3.				
4.				
5.				
6.				
7.				
8.				
9.				
10.				

Once you've filled the left column with the items you usually use, go to each store and write in the appropriate space how much that product costs. When you have completed your chart, highlight the lowest price for each product. Now when you are at each store, you will know what to buy. You might discover that most of the deals are at one particular store. Maybe this is the one to make your primary shopping destination.

You will not shop at each store weekly. You may only shop one or two times per month and stop in for fresh bread, milk, and fresh fruits and vegetables when needed. The key is to stock up on certain items that you know are lower priced on a regular basis at each individual store.

Of course, if another store happens to have something on sale, costing less than I regularly pay for it elsewhere, then I stock up. As I said, shopping this way saves me an estimated 30 percent on average. But for those of us who are busy, this is not always the choice we will make. Shopping at several locations takes more time. We can make more money, but we can't make more time. It's important to be smart with both time and money.

Fighting the Urge to Splurge

Studies show that people who shop with a list spend less money. I suggest a healthy blend of shopping with a list of needed items and also being a smart shopper by being open to the possibility of purchasing sale items if you think you can use them (within the next month for nonperishables and within the week for perishables).

On days when you are not doing your main grocery shopping and are just picking up a few items, taking cash only to the grocery store is a great way to ensure you do not overspend. Haven't we all at one time or another gone into the grocery store to get just a few things and spent a lot more than we intended because we could write a check or charge it?

For small purchases and to help stay focused on getting what you came to purchase, don't get a grocery cart. Pushing a cart makes it easy to purchase extra things you had no intention of buying. If your arms are full carrying the groceries you need, then you are a lot less tempted to grab this and that.

Go to the back of the grocery store and get the heaviest thing first, which is usually milk. A gallon of milk weighs eight pounds. Believe me, carrying that milk vs. putting it in the cart makes the temptation to grab other things a lot less appealing.

When you are doing your main shopping, be careful when going down hard-to-resist aisles. In some cases when there are just too many temptations, I recommend keeping your cart at the end of the aisle, mentally putting blinders on so you are totally focused on exactly what you need to get, and then returning to your cart as quickly as possible. This works for me when I have to go down the cookie aisle. If graham crackers are what I am after, I look straight at my cart to get out of that aisle as fast as I am able so I don't have to hear all those tasty little cookies yelling, "Buy me! Just one little box of these favorite cookies won't hurt. You can get them for the kids!"

If these ideas still aren't enough to help you get through your grocery shopping without buying all kinds of junk food, then I encourage you to ask your spouse, a friend, a neighbor, or a family member if they can pick it up. As you become stronger and more self-confident, then you can test your wings to fly through the grocery store, but in the meantime do what is best for you. That means taking good care of yourself by eliminating temptations rather than trying to resist them.

From Here on Out

The changes you have made and will make are the same things you will need to do to continue being the healthier person you become. Maintenance is extremely important. *Consistency in maintenance is key to lifelong success.*

This concept may be scary and overwhelming for you at first. I encourage you:

You can do it one day at a time. This is going to be a learning process for you. There may be moments you will backslide. That is okay. You are not perfect. Nobody is. Only God is perfect. Don't be hard on yourself. Be gentle, forgiving, and accepting. Treat yourself as you would treat others in your shoes. Strive for perfection, but don't expect perfection. When you make a mistake, pick yourself up, brush yourself off, and start over again.

To reinforce one of our first lessons, your success will happen when you become your biggest supporter. As you extend grace and unconditional love to yourself throughout this process, you might be the first person to give you such goodness ever. God gives this freely, but many women have not been blessed to experience this kind of care from the people in their lives. Be that person for yourself, and soon you will discover that you deserve that kind of treatment from everyone you meet.

The Satisfied Life

"What's in it for me?" "But what do I do next?" "How can I be sure?" These are phrases associated with a dissatisfied life. If they were colors, they would be flashing yellow. Caution. Warning. Do not enter! We say such things to avoid commitment. We use these vague, difficult questions to detract from our lack of answers. But a satisfied life presents a series of statements in place of questions: "God will use this." "I can do great things in this very moment." "Faith will lead me." Commitment is not nearly so scary when we sidestep the questions and go straight for the statements of faith. The satisfied life embraces the certainty of hope and possibility.

Devotional Health

If commitment has not been a strong word in your vocabulary, now is the time to practice repeating that word over and over. Maybe a few of us are commitment-phobes who shy away from signing on the dotted line or writing anything down in pen. You have choices to make. Pray through any concerns you have about committing to your new way of living. Allow God to shed light on the stumbling blocks you may still see as support systems. Write down five things you have already learned about yourself by starting this path of commitment. Write down five things you have learned about God. Keep adding to the list each week. You will be amazed at how many encouraging words are born out of "commitment."

Prayer

Lord, grant me the strength to stay committed to a healthy way of living, thinking, and acting. I long to persevere and need to follow in Your truth to do so. It isn't easy. I want to depend on myself and my emotions to carry me through change and commitment, but You call me to keep my eyes on You and to keep taking one step in front of the other. Thank You for being my source of comfort, inspiration, and identity. Amen.

Complete the Step Seven page of your Personal Plan for a Healthier Me at the back of the book.

The Picture of Health

s your picture of health different now than when you started? Do you have different expectations than when you embarked on previous health journeys? Changing our perspective is as freeing as changing our bad habits into golden ones.

Think about what you want your picture of health to look like. Write it down. Specifically, what do you want your health to feel like, be like? What advantages will it bring to your life? Make a list of how you want to feel physically, spiritually, and emotionally during this journey and as you make progress.

My physical health will look like:

My spiritual health will look like:

My emotional health will look like:

These new pictures of health will keep your goals focused and your motivation high. Instead of cutting out a photo of a skinny model and agonizing over how different your body looks, imagine what *you* would feel like at your optimum health. Consider how optimum health will boost your confidence. Has the idea of it begun to already?

You will discover that doing things light looks easy, manageable, fun, and a lot like the picture of health. Enjoy.

**Step One—Set
Yourself Up for Success**

From my review of programs I have tried or that I have researched, I know that I need _____ and _____ and _____ from a plan. What does not work for me in a program is if that method is _____ and/or _____ _____.

My top three danger zone places to plan around are:

My top three danger zone people to plan around are:

The people in my life who will be most supportive are:

I will support myself by:

**Step Two—Create a
New Relationship with
Food**

My past relationship with food looked a lot like:

My danger zone foods are:

If I look at my calorie count as though it were money, I should be spending $_____ daily.

Go through your book of nutritional information and list

foods you are excited to eat in place of high-risk foods. Try to list as many as you are able so that you have lots of options.

In my health story, I have used food as a:

In my health story, I have sought out food when:

The more I understand that food is meant for fuel and not just for fun and comfort, the more I will be able to:

I plan to save caloric money from now on by:

I am excited about my new relationship with food because:

Step Three—Practice Intentional Eating

From the formula in Step Three, I figured my basal metabolic rate as: _____.

This number is _____ than I expected.

Using the selections in the K.I.S.S. meal plan, my plan for the next week will look like this:

Sample Day:

Breakfast: *French Toast*
Lunch: *Grilled Cheese Sandwich*
Dinner: *Frittata*
Snack(s): *apple, berries*
Freebies: *celery*

Day One:

Breakfast: _____

Lunch: _____

Dinner: _____

Snack(s): _____

Freebies: _____

Day Two:

Breakfast: _____

Lunch: _____

Dinner: _____

Snack(s): _____

Freebies: _____

Day Three:

Breakfast: _____

Lunch: _____

Dinner: _____

Snack(s): _____

Freebies: _____

Day Four:

Breakfast: _____

Lunch: _____

Dinner: _____

Snack(s): _____

Freebies: _____

Day Five:

Breakfast: _____

Lunch: _____

Dinner: _____

Snack(s): _____

Freebies: _____

Day Six:

Breakfast: _____

Lunch: _____

Dinner: _____

Snack(s): _____

Freebies: _____

Day Seven:

Breakfast: _____

Lunch: _____

Dinner: _____

Snack(s): _____

Freebies: _____

My goal is to use the K.I.S.S. plan for _____ weeks to maintain my goal BMR of _____.

Step Four—Move in the Right Direction

Right now my exe

rcise life is (circle one)

Inactive   Moderately active   Very active
                    (3 times a week)   (5 or more
                                              times a week)

Currently I exercise _____ times a week on average.

My usual form of exercise is:

My favorite form of exercise is:

Something I have always wanted to try is:

My goal for this next month is to exercise _____ times a week for _____ minutes.

My schedule for each week could look like this:
(Indicate which days would be "off" and which would be exercise days. It is best if you can put the actual exercise and time in this plan.)

Sunday

Monday

Tuesday

Wednesday

Thursday

Friday

Saturday

Each week I will increase my exercise increments by _____ minutes until I reach one hour at least three times a week.

Someone I will ask to exercise with me is:

This exercise plan is reasonable and something I could stick with because:

Personal Plan for a Healthier Me | Step Five—De-Clutter Your Life

I sense the most clutter is these areas of my life:

I have managed clutter in my home by:

I have managed clutter in my life by:

I have managed clutter in my mind by:

My short to-do list for taking care of clutter in my home is:

In the past, I did not serve my body as a temple when I:

I want to clear away my stinkin' thinking junk food thoughts about healthy foods. Over the next few weeks I will try to trade _____ for a healthier option. And _____ for a healthier food choice.

My five most frequent stinkin' thinking junk food thoughts about my worth that I will clear away are:

1.

2.

3.

4.

5.

I will start to practice easy breathing this week. A good time for me to try it is:

To help me be accountable, I will share my plan for healthier thinking with:

For accountability I will share my plan for healthier eating with:

People I will ask for help in keeping my life less cluttered are (write the names of these people and how you want them to help):

Step Six—Get
Spiritually Fit

I want to be still before God regularly. I will start by spending _____ minutes of time praying and talking to God every _____ at _____.

The three biggest questions I have for God are:

The thing I need to have God do for me because I cannot do it for myself is:

The choices I will make toward spiritual wholeness are:

As I face my lack of will power, I will trust God's will for my life. I experience God's faithfulness in my life in many ways, including:

The verses I want to use as my source of motivation and inspiration for this change are (write them out in full):

Personal Plan for a Healthier Me | Step Seven—Commit to the New Lifestyle

Are you ready to create a specific and realistic plan of action? The more specific your plan of action, the greater your probability for success is. Don't write something vague, such as lose ten pounds. Instead, be specific. Lose ten pounds within eight weeks by:

1. Example: Doing half an hour of aerobic exercise three times a week first thing in the morning from 6:00 to 6:30 AM on Mondays, Wednesdays, and Fridays, and doing toning exercises two days a week from 6:00 to 6:30 AM on Tuesdays and Thursdays. Write your specific exercise plan and at what times you will exercise.

2. Staying away from white flour and white sugar. Write what you're going to stay away from.

3. Eating three small meals of a healthy carbohydrate the size of my fist and lean protein the size of my palm along with up to three snacks daily of no more than 200 calories each and as many fresh green vegetables as I like. Write your eating plan:

4. Eating low-fat, low-sugar foods and drinking sugar-free beverages. Write what danger zone foods and beverages you are going to avoid, and list what you are going to substitute the deleted food with. Example:

replace ice cream at night with one low-fat ice-cream sandwhich.

5. Staying away from processed foods and trying to eat natural foods that God made. List processed junk foods you are going to avoid, and write what healthy choice you are going to substitue. Example: Potato chips for baked potato chips.

6. Getting enough sleep. I will be in bed by _____ daily.

On the following page, create a plan for physical, spiritual, and emotional categories.

Physical Plan of Action

Spiritual Plan of Action

Emotional Plan of Action

Journal Pages

Journal Pages

Journal Pages

Journal Pages

Journal Pages

Journal Pages

Journal Pages

Journal Pages

Journal Pages

Journal Pages

Journal Pages

Journal Pages

Journal Pages

Journal Pages

Journal Pages

Journal Pages

Journal Pages

Journal Pages

How to Contact the Author

Dawn Hall is the award-winning author of *Down Home Cookin' Without the Down Home Fat, Busy People's Low-Fat Cookbook, Busy People's Slow Cooker Cookbook, Busy People's Diabetic Cookbook, Busy People's Low-Carb Cookbook,* and *Busy People's Christmas Cookbook.*

She is also the host of *Cooking for Busy People,* a 30-minute television show aired nationally. As a popular inspirational speaker, Dawn brings hope and healing to audiences across the country.

To communicate with Dawn about speaking engagements, please contact her at:

dawn@dawnhallcookbooks.com

5425 Fulton-Lucas Rd.
Swanton, OH 43558
Phone: (419) 826–2665
Fax: (419) 825–2700

Discover more about Dawn, her books,
and her speaking ministry by visiting her website:

www.dawnhallcookbooks.com

Other Good Harvest House Reading

Overcoming Runaway Blood Sugar
By Dennis Pollock
After author Dennis Pollock experienced a serious diabetic episode, he created a succesful program to normalize blood sugar levels. He shares how to remove risks for blood sugar irregularities and how to achive optimum health.

Balance That Works When Life Doesn't
By Susie Larson
Life sometimes seems out of control. How can women possibly balance all the demands of a Christian lifestyle? Susie Larson invites you to effectively respond and adjust to the opportunities and assignments God gives you.

BASIC Steps to Godly Fitness
By Laurette Willis
In this uniquely integrated program, certified personal trainer and aerobic instructor Laurette Willis shares her BASIC (Body And Soul In Christ), step-by-step plan to improve wholeness in body, soul, and spirit.

Greater Health God's Way
By Stormie Omartian
For everyone who has tried diet programs, only to find them less than completely satisfying, bestselling author Stormie Omartian provides a creative, practical approach to developing a person's mind, body, and spirit by outlining seven steps to a healthy life.

Love to Eat, Hate to Eat
By Elyse Fitzpatrick
After years of futile dieting, readers know there's more to weight control than what they eat. Having discovered the power that food has over their lives, counselor Elyse Fitzpatrick helps them in their battle of the bulge.